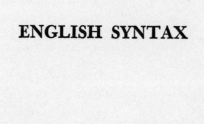

ENGLISH SYNTAX

ENGLISH SYNTAX

An Outline for Clinicians and Teachers
of Language Handicapped Children

By

CHARLES H. HARGIS

*Professor, Department of Special
Education and Rehabilitation
The University of Tennessee
Knoxville, Tennessee*

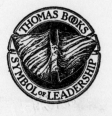

CHARLES C THOMAS · PUBLISHER
Springfield · Illinois · U.S.A.

Published and Distributed Throughout the World by
CHARLES C THOMAS • PUBLISHER
BANNERSTONE HOUSE
301-327 East Lawrence Avenue, Springfield, Illinois, U.S.A.

© *1977, by* CHARLES C THOMAS • PUBLISHER
ISBN 0-398-03558-X
Library of Congress Catalog Card Number: 76-3575

Printed in the United States of America
N-1

Library of Congress Cataloging in Publication Data

Hargis, Charles H.
    English syntax.

    Bibliography: p.
    Includes index.
    1. English language—Study and teaching (Primary) 2. English
language—Syntax. 3. English language—Grammar, Generative. I. Title.
LB1528.H34   371.9'14   76-3575
ISBN 0-398-03558-X

PREFACE

L ANGUAGE BASICALLY has three components—its vocabulary or lexicon, its figurative devices and its syntax. Of the three, syntax appears most to be a function of developmental readiness levels when children acquire language. This acquisitive process appears to parallel and even reflect the cognitive development described by Piaget. The acquisition of syntax is largely complete in the majority of nonhandicapped children by about age seven or about the end of Piaget's preoperational period of cognitive development. More crucial, though, to this developmental notion of the acquisition of syntax is the evidence, especially noted by Eric Lenneberg, that the acquisition of syntax is subject to critical readiness periods after which normal acquisition processes are severely curtailed. The normal readiness period for syntax acquisition appears to end with the advent of adolescence. Subsequently, this relatively short time period that the normal language learning mechanisms are operative suggests that a most expeditious form of education or remediative attention be directed to the development of syntax in children whose normal acquisition processes are impeded or delayed by severe forms of language deprivation, primarily hearing impairments, or by central nervous system dysfunction.

It must be pointed out that the knowledge of syntax of children is not of the conscious type. This knowledge is not of the name and function of the various syntactic structures to use in communication, but it is the intuitive knowledge available to all nonhandicapped persons which permits them to understand any and all syntactic forms and to produce them. However, it is just this sort of conscious knowledge of syntax that is necessary for the teacher or clinician who intends to work with language handicapped children. The more adequate and detailed this knowledge, the more adequte and detailed may be the diagnosis and prescription for the handicapped child. More specifically, the teacher or clinician should be able to accurately identify any child's level of syntactic development, then provide curricular materials suited to his needs on a developmental continuum.

The scope of syntax covered in this book is intended to include as much as possible what the normal child acquires during the age period from two to seven. All of the structures contained in this outline are used in the language of popular first grade level basal reading series. The author has personally analyzed the popular basal readers and has reported these findings (Hargis, 1974). This fact emphasizes the need for mastery of syntax before a child is prepared for normal achievement entry into regular school curricula.

The method of description and analysis of the syntactic structures in the book is that of the transformational generative grammar. The theoretical basis for each structure and transformation is not dealt with, only the description and analysis. The approach does not assume previous knowledge of this system, but it does presuppose that the reader accept it as an adequate descriptive and analytic method.

After the material is covered, the final two chapters illustrate some methods of assessing a child's mastery of syntax and some teaching materials and methods.

ACKNOWLEDGMENTS

I wish to express my appreciation for the assistance of some of my former students in the preparation of this manuscript. They are Karen Piazza, Cathy Crossland Mahmoud and Diane Karides Hudson.

C.H.H.

CONTENTS

ENGLISH SYNTAX

INTRODUCTION

KNOWLEDGE OF SYNTAX

W HEN A CHILD'S HANDICAPPING CONDITION is most clearly defined in terms of a language deficiency, the teacher or clinician who works with such a child requires a thorough knowledge of the constructs of language. This knowledge is requisite to the adequate diagnosis of each child's language comprehension and production ability. The clinician or teacher will be required to identify the child's specific level of performance. This is necessary to identify the language readiness level or entry level in the scope and sequence of language components which comprise the essential features of English. The teacher or clinician must be aware of the scope of essentials of the language that a normal child learns from about age two to about age seven. The focus of this book is the syntax which the normal child acquires during this time period.

The clinician must have a sufficient knowledge of syntax to be able to diagnostically construct the child's grammar and work within it. By constructing this grammar the clinician can identify the communication threshold within which and through which a language program or curriculum can be prescribed. Also, by working within this threshold or readiness level the clinician is able to provide adequate manageable instructional materials which are not failure inducing. A comprehensive knowledge of syntactic structure is necessary to evaluate the structure of existing materials or to prepare materials for use with children according to their level of syntactic functioning. The clinician must be prepared to program systematically the syntactic elements which have been diagnosed as missing, with the ultimate objective as mastery of the syntax of English.

This knowledge of syntax is necessary for the teacher to be able to impose an external organization on syntactic input to expedite or facilitate its learning. This external organization is needed to help bypass the obstruction to syntactic acquisition imposed by defective auditory or perceptual channels. It may also be necessary to bypass or traverse some central nervous system dysfunction. Normal children can impose their internal organizational structures and perceptual processes on the relatively unorganized language stimulation available in the environment and quite adequately acquire language. The external organization in the curriculum is intended to make up for the defective internal organizational structures or perceptual processes of the language handicapped child.

CRITICAL READINESS PERIODS

The precise boundaries of the age range for the acquisition of syntax are not yet available. Current literature (Palermo and Molfese, 1972) suggests that acquisition processes likely extend considerably further than age five which was formerly felt to represent roughly the boundary for completion. However, Lenneberg (1967) ties the acquisition of syntax to the age range from two to twelve. Age twelve represents the upper limit after which the capacity for primary language synthesis is lost. Hargis, Mercaldo and Johnson (1975) review and point to the sequential nature of the acquisition process and how a child may be fixed or cut off at a point on this development continuum with the advent of adolescence or the end of the critical readiness period. A recent study reported by Curtiss, Fromkin, Krashen and Rigler (1974) indicates the tragic results of extreme language deprivation throughout the critical period in a normal child. Less dramatic, but nonetheless significant, information concerns second language learning before, during, and after adolescence. This information is more and more frequently reported by linguists interested in foreign language instruction.

The fact of critical readiness periods must influence the calendar applied to language curriculum and instructional strategies. Also, the problem of postadolescent language learning will likely necessitate the use and development of even more robust language intervention techniques for older students.

LANGUAGE AND COGNITION

The relationship of language to thought has a long history of philosophical interest. However, Piaget (1969) and Furth (1966) point out the functioning of thought or cognition without language. Piaget discusses the possibility of concrete operational thought without language but describes the necessity of language as a necessary component in formal operational thought (cognitive processes which develop after approximately age 11). Hargis et al. (1975) point to the primary relation of cognitive structure to language through the operational levels (ages 2 through 11). Cognitive structures and the level of cognitive development of a child represent the readiness base for the acquisition of each syntactic structure which can map it into a communication act.

The sequence of development of cognitive structure provides a guide to the scope and sequence of many syntactic structures. Some of the following chapters are prepared so as to better illustrate the syntactic organization of some important cognitive areas. A further point needs to be made concerning the cognitive-linguistic relationship. Any language development program should firmly tie the learning of syntactic forms to the appropriate conceptual experience and assure that the language intervention level is within the cognitive readiness level of each child. Conceptual development is primary in order.

DEVELOPMENTAL HANDICAPPING CONDITIONS

Very generally, developmental language handicapping conditions are of three types. The first type includes hearing impairments with ages of onset and degrees which reduce language stimulation to levels that preclude the normal development of syntactic forms as maps of the normally acquired cognitive structures. The second is central nervous systems dysfunctions which impair the activity of the language acquisition devices (Chomsky, 1965) that are engaged in organizing auditory language input and mapping it onto emerging cognitive structures. The third type consists of mental retardation of nonfamilial types. Familial retardates with an IQ 50 or above can be expected to have normal, if somewhat delayed, language development (Hargis et al., 1975). Children with IQ's below 50 will have more pronounced language deficiencies as the intelligence level declines below 50. In the case of the nonfamilial retardation, the problem of language acquisition is directly related to missing cognitive structure. There can be no linguistic map for a nonexistent cognitive structure. Language programs for these children must direct primary attention to each child's level of cognitive development. This level of development may suggest their readiness for language learning as well as the concepts and experiences which will necessarily precede the next level of language attainment. The language functioning of these children may be most useful described in terms of the stage of operational level of cognitive attainment.

COMPREHENSION AND PRODUCTION

Chomsky's (1965) theoretical work concerns an ideal speaker-listener in a homogeneous speech community. This person has a complete intuitive mastery of the language (competence) and is able to use it in listening and speaking situations (performance) at an equally high level. This idealized person is not troubled by the memory limitations of ordinary people nor any impairments that face the exceptional. Chomsky's purpose in describing this person was for explaining the parameters of the most complete grammar of a language possible. Chomsky was, however, well aware of the practical distinctions between the ideal speaker-listener and real life speaker-listener.

The real world performance problems of exceptional children are the concern of teachers and clinicians. The performance categories of language comprehension and production are the scope for the assessments and interventions by teachers and clinicians.

Linguistic studies (McNeill, 1966, 1970; Brown and Bellugi, 1964; Menyuk, 1969; among others) point to a sequential progression that children follow as they master the grammar of their language. However, McNeill points out that the language comprehension of children both precedes and exceeds substantially their productive ability. The majority of normal children, when they are ready to begin school, can usually comprehend and enjoy a wide variety of children's literature and can comprehend and follow rather complex directions for a variety of games and activities. However, when the same children attempt to tell a story or to give directions, their production attempts are characterized by considerable dysfluency. The sequence of events may be disarranged. There will be many false starts and hesitations. This normal discrepancy between comprehension and production may be more notable at these early ages, but it does seem to persist into adulthood with, of course, considerable individual levels of difference.

The comprehension-production distinction is a very important fact to keep in mind for both diagnosis and language programming. The diagnostician must not overly rely on production information to give evidence of level of comprehension. Also, fluent expressive ability cannot be expected to match a child's level of comprehension. In language programming the production aspect will likely require activities specific to its development. Because a child acquires the comprehension of a linguistic structure does not mean that it would be immediately and easily available in his or her expressive ability. The expressive use of the structure may well be on a different developmental timetable.

ORGANIZATION OF THE BOOK

The book's organization is intended to assist in achieving several objectives. The first objective is to provide a practical outline of the essential features of English syntax for use by teachers and clinicians. The second purpose is didactic. The organization is intended to assist the person who has no formal training in linguistics to acquire a conscious operational knowledge of the workings of English syntax for use in the classroom or clinical setting. At the end of most topical chapters there are review exercises which are intended to assist in mastery. The third purpose is to provide information on application. The final two chapters attempt to relate the topic areas to assessment and intervention techniques.

SENTENCE CLASSES

F UNDAMENTALLY, language is comprised of a number of elementary sentence types. These basic sentences are the underlying source of all of the more complex sentences which can be produced.

There are some distinctions and differences between these elementary sentence types. The differences and the descriptions of the various elementary sentence classes are probably best defined by the verbs or verb phrases used in them. All of these sentences (S) contain a subject noun phrase (NP), an auxiliary (Aux) and a verb phrase (VP). This description of a sentence is frequently written as the phrase structure rule,

$$S \longrightarrow NP + AUX + VP$$

The nature and constituent structure of the noun phrase and auxiliary will receive specific detailed treatment in subsequent chapters. The verb phrase will be expanded in connection with embedding transformations to be discussed later. For the purpose of developing the foundation perspective provided by an understanding of these simple sentences, the following general descriptions are important.

INTRANSITIVE VERBS (VI)

The simple sentences constituting this class are formed by a subject and a verb:

1. The baby crawls.
2. The boy walks.
3. The roof leaks.

Intransitive verbs will not be followed by either an adjective

8

or noun. Some intransitive verbs, such as hang, stay, live, etc., must be followed by adverbs:

4. The picture hangs *on the wall*.
5. The man stayed *at home*.
6. The girl lives *on a farm*.

TRANSITIVE VERBS (VT)

The verbs in this sentence class are followed by noun phrases known as direct objects:

1. They hid *the cookies*.
2. A man bought *a book*.

Some transitive verbs can be followed by an indirect object as well as the direct object. The prepositional phrase form of the indirect object will usually begin with the prepositions *to* or *for* and will follow the direct object. The nonprepositional forms of the indirect objects will precede the direct object:

3. Joe gave the ball to Fred.
4. The man bought a bike for the boy.
5. Joe gave *Fred* the ball.
6. The man bought *the boy* a bike.

Transitive verbs that require an animate object, such as *surprise* and *please,* cannot take indirect objects:

7. The boy surprised the skunk.
8. The child pleased the teacher.

At least one transitive verb, *put,* seems to require an adverb of place following the direct object in order to be grammatical:

9. He put the bike *in the garage*.
10. He put the roast *in the oven*.

COPULATIVE VERBS

All of the copulative verb forms share at least one common feature. This minimum commonality is that they can be followed by an adjective.

BE. The sentences containing *be* as the verb have a variety of different forms. *Be* may be followed by an adjective:

1. The boy is *tall*.
2. The girl was *happy*.

Be can be followed by a noun phrase:
   3. The man is *an Indian*.
   4. The plane was *a jet*.

It can be followed by an adverb of place:
   5. The bird is *in a tree*.
   6. The boy is *at home*.

Be can be followed by *for* plus a nominal form:
   7. The gift is *for you*.
   8. The wrench is *for the machine*.

Be can be followed by *like* plus a nominal form:
   9. The language was *like Russian*.
  10. The wood is *like walnut*.

STAY AND REMAIN. The sentences comprising this subset of copulative verb types seem to share many of the same forms as *be* sentences. When they are used as copulative verbs, they may be followed by an adjective.
  11. The child stayed *happy*.
  12. The shrubs remained *small*.

They can be followed by a noun phrase:
  13. John remained *the secretary*.
  14. The Indian stayed *chief*.

They may be followed by an adverb of place:
  15. Fred stayed *at home*.
  16. One bird remained *in the tree*.

Stay and *remain* can be followed by *like* plus a nominal form:
  17. Fred remains *like his father*.
  18. The boy stayed *like a child*.

BECOME. Sentences of this copulative form may be followed by adjectives, noun phrases or *like* plus a nominal form. Consider the examples respectively:
  19. The boy became *ill*.
  20. The boy became a *man*.

21. The boy became like his *father*.

APPEAR. This class commonly includes *seem* and *look*. These verbs of appearance in their simplest forms may be followed by adjectives, or *like* plus a nominal form:

22. She seems *happy*.
23. They look *silly*.
24. They look *like flowers*.

SENSE VERBS (VS)

This class includes the verbs *taste, smell, feel,* etc. These verbs are followed by adjectives or *like* plus a nominal form:

25. The punch tasted *sweet*.
26. The carpet felt *rough*.
27. The flower smelled *good*.
28. The floor felt *like sandpaper*.

GROW AND TURN. This class of sentences contains action verbs such as *grow* or *turn* in their copulative form. These verbs will be followed by adjectives:

29. The milk turned *sour*.
30. The man grew *old*.

HAVE

This sentence class contains the verb forms *have, cost* and *weigh* which share the syntactic characteristics of being followed only by a noun phrase and of having no passive forms. However, semantically the *have* verbs generally convey some notion of possession while the *cost* and *weigh* verbs are restricted to indication of quantity or amount:

1. The boy has *a dog*.
2. The boys weighs *seventy pounds*.
3. The pot costs *five dollars*.

CHANGES IN VERB CLASS

Many verbs, including some of those described above, may not always appear in the same sentence or verb class. For example, the intransitive verb *walk* can be used as a transitive verb:

1. The boy walked. (intransitive)
2. The boy walked the dog. (transitive)

Some of the copulative verb forms have transitive uses:

3. Fred turned pale. (copulative)
4. Fred turned the eggs. (transitive)
5. The milk tasted sour. (copulative)
6. John tasted the milk. (transitive)

PROBLEMS WITH SIMPLE SENTENCE FORMS

The terms *elementary* or *simple* were just used to describe various basic sentence classes. These terms were not intended to mask the conceptual or syntactic difficulty that these structures may pose in language acquisition. The problems with acquisition of these elementary sentence forms are in both comprehension and production.

COMPREHENSION PROBLEMS. *Have* and *be* sentences constitute probably the most common classes, but they also pose some confusing problems to the handicapped child (Hargis and Lamm, 1974). *Have* generally indicates possession; however it has semantic subclassifications which may require specific individual attention. Some of these subsets are:

1. I have two arms. (body parts)
2. Fred has a pencil. (immediate ownership)
3. Fred has Mary's book. (temporary possession)
4. Joe has a book at home. (remote ownership)

The notion of possession is not made uniform by the use of the common verb *have*. Body parts are a systemic element (sent. 1), but you can own something not attached to you (sent. 2). You can also own something you cannot see (sent. 4). Further, you may have something that you don't own (sent. 3). Each of these subclassifications may require conceptual organization to facilitate acquisition.

The sense verb *feel* may pose an early comprehension problem when the distinction must be made between the concrete tactual notion of how things feel (sent. 7, 8):

5. The floor feels rough.

6. The blanket feels smooth.
7. Mary feels sick.
8. Joe feels angry.

PRODUCTION PROBLEMS. The most serious production problems will likely occur because of the confusion that results from superficial resemblance of *have* and *be* sentence forms. Both verbs can be followed by a noun phrase. Errors caused by this confusion are commonly noted in the expressive language of congenitally deaf children. Errors such as the following have been noted:

*9. I am brown eyes.
*10. My eyes have brown.
*11. Fred has a sick.
*12. Joe is a sick.
*13. Joe is a flu.

These children may be confusing the form of *be* which is followed by an adjective with the form where it is followed by a noun phrase. Because *have* is followed by a noun phrase, these children might think that all of the forms are interchangeable. The inappropriate use of an article with an adjective and a noun, for either may appear after the *be* verb.

AGREEMENT. The production difficulties related to tense and number agreement are viewed as problems related to memory and rote or associative learning. This is especially true for the learning of the high frequency irregular verb forms. Rule learning likely occurs after the child has a sufficient stock of regular verb forms from which to generalize.

THE AUXILIARY

I N THE PRECEDING chapter this phrase structure rule for sentences was presented:

$$S \longrightarrow NP + AUX + VP$$

The VP was the focus of attention as a set of elementary sentences was described. The auxiliary (AUX) will be the focus of attention over this and the next chapter. The phrase structure rule for the auxiliary which will be discussed in this chapter is Noam Chomsky's (1957) well-known formulation:

$$AUX \longrightarrow Tense + (Modal) + (have+en) + (being)$$

In this description the parenthesis means that the element need not be present in the auxiliary, but any combination of elements must follow the indicated order. Notice that *tense* is the only element which is not enclosed by parenthesis. Tense must appear in the auxiliary.

Before we can further illustrate, the auxiliary components must be elaborated. The first of these is *tense,* which is composed of *present* or *past*:

$$Tense \longrightarrow Present, Past$$

The second description is for the *modal,* which traditionally was thought to be composed of will, can, may, shall, must:

$$Modal \longrightarrow will, can, may, shall, must$$

The verb forms be, have, VT, VI and VS are used in all of the following sentence examples to illustrate the various auxiliary combinations.

TENSE

Tense will always occur in the auxiliary of a sentence. The following simple sentences contain present tense in their auxiliaries:

14

(be)   1. NP + present + be +
         adj   The girl is happy.

(have)   2. NP + present + have +
         NP   The boy has a dog.

(VT)   3. NP + present + make +
         NP   Mother makes a cake.

(VI)   4. NP + present + run   The dog runs.

(VS)   5. NP + present + taste +
         adj   The milk tastes sour.

The following sentences contain past tense in their auxiliaries:

1. NP + past + be + adj   The girl was happy.
2. NP + past + have + NP The boy had a dog.
3. NP + past + run   The dog ran.
4. NP + past + make + NP Mother made a cake.
5. NP + past + taste + adj The milk tasted sour.

Notice how tense joins the verb form which follows it. This joining or affixing produces both the regular and irregular past tense forms of verbs.

MODALS

In addition to present tense, the following simple sentences contain modals in their auxiliaries:

1. NP + present + will +
   be + adj   The girl *will* be happy.
2. NP + present + can +
   have + NP   The boy *can* have a dog.
3. NP + present + shall +
   make + NP   Mother *shall* make a cake.
4. NP + present + may +
   run   The dog *may* run.
5. NP + present + must +
   taste + adj   The milk *must* taste sour.

HAVE + EN

The auxiliary structure (have+en) forms are traditionally called the *perfect* tenses. The parenthesis indicate that the two elements constitute a single unit. They must occur together. Notice how *en* is affixed to the following verbs, producing various *past participle* forms in the sentence examples. The following examples contain the sequence present tense plus (have+en) in their auxiliaries:

1. NP + present + (have+en) +
   be + adj   The girl has been happy.
2. NP + present + (have+en) +
   have + NP   The boy has had a dog.
3. NP + present + (have+en) +
   make + NP   Mother has made a cake.
4. NP + present + (have+en) +
   run   The dog has run.
5. NP + present + (have+en) +
   taste + adj   The milk has tasted sour.

These examples contain past tense plus (have+en) in their auxiliaries:

1. NP + past + (have+en) +
   be + adj   The girl had been happy.
2. NP + past + (have+en) +
   have + NP   The boy had had a dog.
3. NP + past + (have+en) +
   make + NP   Mother had made a cake.
4. NP + past + (have+en) +
   run   The dog had run.
5. NP + past + (have+en) +
   taste + adj   The milk had tasted sour.

BE + ING

The auxiliary structure (be+ing) represents what is traditionally called the *progressive* tense. Again, as with (have+en), the parenthesis indicates that the two elements constitute a single auxiliary element. They must occur together. The *ing* element is affixed to the verb forms that follow it. The following examples represent the sequence present tense plus (be+ing) in the auxiliary:

1. NP + present + (be+ing) +
   be + adj   The girl is being happy.
2. NP + present + (be+ing) +
   have + NP   The boy is having fun.
3. NP + present + (be+ing) +
   make + NP   Mother is making a cake.
4. NP + present + (be+ing) +
   run   The dog is running.
5. NP + present + (be+ing) +
   taste + adj   The milk is tasting sour.

The next examples illustrate the auxiliary sequence past tense plus (be+ing) :

1. NP + past + (be+ing) +
   be + adj   The girl was being happy.
2. NP + past + (be+ing) +
   have + NP   The boy was having fun.
3. NP + past + (be+ing) +
   make + NP   Mother was making a cake.
4. NP + past + (be+ing) +
   run   The dog was running.
5. NP + past + (be+ing) +
   taste + adj   The milk was tasting sour.

AUXILIARY COMBINATIONS

The various sentence examples presented so far have shown simple auxiliaries and simple combinations of auxiliary structures. However, the elements of the auxiliary can be used in more complex combinations. The following examples will illustrate the combinations possible from the auxiliary formula:

Aux ⟶ Tense + (Modal) + (have+en) + (be+ing)

Aux ⟶ Tense + (Modal) + (have+en) . Three auxiliary elements are used in these examples. Notice how tense (present or past) and participle (en) influence the words which follow them:

1. NP + past + will +   The girl would have been
   (have+en) + be + adj   happy.

2. NP + past + may +
(have+en) + have + NP
The boy might have had a dog.

3. NP + past + can +
(have+en) + make + NP
Mother could have made a cake.

4. NP + present + shall +
(have+en) + run
The dog shall have run.

5. NP + present + must +
(have+en) + taste + adj
The milk must have tasted sour.

AUX ———→ TENSE + (MODAL) + (BE+ING). Three auxiliary elements are used in these examples also:

1. NP + past + will +
(be+ing) + be + adj
The girl would be being happy.

2. NP + past + may +
(be+ing) + have + NP
The boy might be having fun.

3. NP + past + can +
(be+ing) + make + NP
Mother could be making a cake.

4. NP + present +
(have+en) + (be+ing)
+ run
The dog has been running.

5. NP + present +
(have+en) + (be+ing)
+ taste + adj
The milk has been tasting sour.

AUX ———→ TENSE + (MODAL) + (HAVE+EN) + (BE+ING). In each of these examples, all four auxiliary elements are used:

1. NP + past + will +
(have+en) + (be+ing)
+ be + adj
The girl would have been being happy.

2. NP + past + will +
(have+en) + (be+ing)
+ be + adj
The boy would have been having fun.

3. NP + past + can +
(have+en) + (be+ing)
+ make + NP
Mother could have been making a cake.

4. NP + present + shall +
(have+en) + (be+ing)
+ run
The dog should have been running.

5. NP + present + must +   The milk must have been
(have+en) + (be+ing)   tasting sour.
+ taste + adj

ADDITIONAL MODAL FORMS

The five modals, *will, can, may, shall* and *must,* were introduced and illustrated in sentence examples in this chapter. *Need* and *dare* are sometimes called semimodals. They are used infrequently. Each has a much more common verb form. Recent work on modals in English (Hakutani and Hargis, 1972) expands this class to include the more common forms *ought to, used to, had better* and *had best.* The additional members of the modal category are illustrated in the following examples:

1. NP + tense + ought to   The girl *ought to* be hap-
+ be + adj   py.
2. NP + tense + used to   The boy *used to* have fun.
+ have + NP
3. NP + tense + had better   Mother *had better* make a
+ make + NP   cake.
4. NP + tense + had best   The dog *had best* run.
+ run

There appears to be only one tense form for *used to, had better* and *had best. Ought to* is synonymous with the traditional modal *should.*

PRESENT TENSE

The simple present tense form of verbs—that is, when only present tense occurs in the auxiliary—may pose special conceptual problems. The simple present tense form can be used to state generalizations or to indicate habitual states:

1. Birds fly.
2. Beavers build dams.
3. Farmers grow crops.
4. Elephants are strong.

The *present progressive tense* represented by present tense plus *be+ing* in the auxiliary *is* used to indicate current ongoing activity.

HAVE + EN

The auxiliary element *have+en* is probably the most difficult auxiliary component. Present tense plus *have+en*, the present perfect tense, implies an occurrence in an unspecified prior past period. Past tense plus *have+en*, the past perfect tense, implies an occurrence completed in a prior past period with an intervening occurrence. Consider the following examples:

1. The patient has died.
2. The patient had died *by the time the doctor arrived*.

The rather complex time relationships imposed by *have+en* in the auxiliary may account for the difficulty. Paula Menyuk, who has done extensive work in language acquisition (1964, 1969), indicates that normal children in the age range from five to seven years still do not show complete development of *have* in the auxiliary.

REVIEW EXERCISES

The following exercises cover the various auxiliary elements presented in the chapter. The exercise is on the left-hand side of the page and the answer for each numbered item is placed next to it on the right hand side of the page.

1. A girl + present + will
   + walk

   A girl will walk.

2. The boy + past +
   (be+ing) + run

   The boy was running.

3. The candy + past +
   (have+en) + taste +
   good

   The candy had tasted good.

4. The boy + present +
   will + (be+ing) + go

   The boy will be going.

5. The pig + past + may
   + (have+en) + be + big

   The pig might have been big.

6. A plant + present +
   must + have + water

   A plant must have water.

7. The lady + past + can +
   (have+en) + (be+ing)
   + buy + the coat

   The lady could have been buying the coat.

8. John + past + shall +
   (have+en) + (be+ing)
   + study

   John should have been studying.

9. The child + present +
   must + (have+en) +
   (be+ing) + eat + some
   candy

   The child must have been eating some candy.

10. The apple + past + can
    + (have+en) + have
    + a worm

    The apple could have had a worm.

Expand the auxiliary of the following two sentences:

A. Birds fly.

1. NP + past + (be+ing)
   + VI

   Birds were flying.

2. NP + present +
   (have+en) + VI

   Birds have been flying.

3. NP + present + will +
   (have+en) + (be+ing)
   + VI

   Birds will have been flying.

B. The cat catches mice.

1. NP + past + VT + NP

   The cat caught mice.

2. NP + present +
   (have+en) + (be+ing)
   + VT + NP

   The cat has been catching mice.

3. NP + past + can +
   (have+en) + VT + NP

   The cat could have caught mice.

4. NP + past + shall +
   (have+en) + (be+ing)
   + catch + NP

   The cat should have been catching mice.

CHAPTER 4

THE AUXILIARY CONTINUED

I N THE PRECEDING CHAPTER the basic auxiliary rule was presented:

Aux———→ Tense + (Modal) + (have+en) + (be+ing)

This rule requires slight alteration to account for some common structures which are found frequently in the language of children. For example, children will use the structures *have to* and *be going to* much more regularly than their nearly synonymous forms *must* and *will:*

1. I *must* go.
2. I *have to* go.
3. I *will* go.
4. I *am going to* go.

Structures like *have to* and *be going to* are called quasi-modals or symbolically stated simply Q. *Have to* and *be going to* are the most common quasi-modals. The class of quasi-modals also includes *be about to, be to, be able to* and *be unable to.* Consider the following examples with these quasi-modals in the auxiliaries of each sentence:

5. He *is about to* go.
6. They *are to* go.
7. He *is able to* go.
8. They *are unable to* go.

We also find that these quasi-modals can be used with considerably more flexibility than the regular modals. The regular modals are confined to the slot immediately following tense in the auxiliary. In most dialects only one regular modal can be used per auxiliary. However, the quasi-modal (Q) does not operate under the same constraints. We find that more than one Q can appear in an auxiliary:

9. Joe *is going to have to go.* (Joe + present + (Q) + (Q) + go)

Q's can appear between other auxiliary elements as in this common sentence:

10. Joe has *had to* work hard. (Joe + present + (have+en) + (Q) + work + hard)

Notice that if we attempt to use the synonymous regular modal in place of the Q's in the two previous examples, the sentences will not be acceptable:

*11. Joe will must go.

*12. Joe has must work hard.

The Q's *be able to* and *be unable to* have one restriction on their use. Both require an animate subject. The regular modal *can* will be used with inanimate subjects:

*13. A chair is able to feel hard.

14. A chair can feel hard.

*15. The hammer is unable to remove the nail.

16. The hammer cannot remove the nail.

THE ELABORATED AUXILIARY RULE

The auxiliary rule must account for the flexibility of quasi-modal constructions. It must account for the Q's repeatability and the fact that they can follow any auxiliary element, including a regular modal. The rule that was developed to account for Q's (Hakutani and Hargis, 1972), is

$$\text{Aux} \longrightarrow \text{Tense} + (\text{Modal}) + (Q)^n + (\text{have+en}) + (Q)^n + (\text{be+ing}) + (Q)^n$$

The exponent n by each quasi-modal slot simply indicates that Q's may be repeated. The first element in all of the quasi-modal forms accepts whatever affix is supplied from tense, *en* or *ing*. The first element will also change according to subject agreement requirements. Each quasi-modal ends in the infinitive marker *to*, thereby leaving any following auxiliary element or verb uninflected.

The following illustration of the elaborated auxiliary rule presents the quasi-modal in the various possible positions and combinations.

Aux⟶ Tense + (Q). The illustrations here show *tense* and Q in the auxiliary:

1. NP + present + (have to) + be + adj   The girl has to be happy.

2. NP + past + (be going to) + have + NP   The boy was going to have fun.

3. NP + past + (be about to) + make + NP   Mother was about to make a cake.

Aux⟶ Tense + (Modal) + (Q). In these examples, Q's follow regular modals:

4. NP + present + will + (be unable to) + run   The dog will be unable to run.

5. NP + past + will + (have to) + taste + sour   The lemons would have to taste sour.

6. NP + past + shall + (be able to) + be + NP   The girl should be able to be a doctor.

Aux⟶ Tense + (Q) (have+en). These examples show Q's preceding *have+en* in the auxiliary:

7. NP + present + (have to) + have+en) + have + NP   The boy has to have had fun.

8. NP + past + (be able to) + (have+en) + make + NP   Mother was able to have made a cake.

9. NP + past + (have to) + (have-+en) + taste + adj   The lemons had to have tasted sour.

Aux⟶ Tense + (Q) + (be+ing). Q's precede *be+ing* in the auxiliary in these examples:

10. NP + past +   Mother was going to be
    (be going to) + (be+ing)   making a cake.
    + make + NP

11. NP + past +   The dog was about to be
    (be about to) + (be+ing)   running.
    + run

12. NP + present +   The girl has to be being
    (have to) + (be+ing)   good.
    + be + adj

Aux⟶ Tense + (be+ing) + (Q). The Q's beginning
with *be* do not occur as readily or naturally after *be+ing*. The
restrictions here are due to the semantic, not syntactic, nature of
those Q's.

13. NP + past + (be+ing)   The boy was having to be
    + (have to) +   good.
    be + adj

14. NP + past + (be+ing)   Mother was being about
    + (be about to) +   to make a cake.
    make + NP

15. NP + present + (be+ing)   The dog is being unable
    + (be unable to) + run   to run.

Aux⟶ Tense + (Q)^n. In these examples, repetition of
Q's is illustrated. Although indefinite repetition of Q's is theoreti-
cally permissible, the performance limitation of memory storage
and processing prevents it. These same performance limitations
prevent the comprehension of all overly complex but gramatically
acceptable utterances. Consider these examples with the double
and triple occurrence of Q:

16. NP + present +   The dog is going to have
    (be going to) +   to run.
    (have to) + run

17. NP + past + (have to)   Mother had to be able
    + (be able to) +   to make a cake.
    make + NP

18. NP + present +　　　　　　The boy is going to be
　　 (be going to) +　　　　　　unable to go.
　　 (be unable to) + go

19. NP + past + (be to)　　　　Joe was to have to be
　　 + (have to) +　　　　　　 about to go.
　　 (be about to) + go

Aux ———→ Tense + (Q) + (HAVE+EN) + (Q). The examples
Q's are used in the auxiliary on either side of *have+en:*

20. NP + present + (have to)　　The boy has to have
　　 + (have+en) +　　　　　　been able to work.
　　 (be able to) + work

21. NP + past + (be about to)　 Mother was about to have
　　 + (have+en) + (have to)　　had to make a cake.
　　 + make + (a cake)

Aux ———→ Tense + (Q) + (BE+ING) + (Q). The examples
illustrate Q's, both before and after *be+ing:*

22. NP + past + (be to)　　　　Joe was to be having
　　 + (be+ing) + (have to)　　 to drive.
　　 + drive

23. NP + present +　　　　　　Fred is about to be
　　 (be about to) +　　　　　 having to find to job.
　　 (be+ing) + (have to)
　　 + find + NP

Aux———→ Tense + (Modal) + (Q) + (HAVE+EN) +
(Q) + (BE+ING) + (Q). Consider these final examples where
three quasi-modals are used according to the formula. The first
example will be without the regular modal, and the second example will be with the regular modal. Remember the language
performance limitations make the likelihood of such structures
very remote.

24. NP + past + (be to) +　　　The winner was to have
　　 (have+en) + (be going to)　been going to be having
　　 + (be+ing) + (have to) +　 to accept the prize.
　　 accept + NP

25. NP + present + (will)　　　 The dog will have to have
　　 + (have to) + (have+en)　　been going to be having
　　 + (be going to) +　　　　 to run.
　　 (be+ing) + (have to) + run

REVIEW EXERCISES

Rewrite the following formula into sentence forms. In this set of exercises, let Q = *have to.*

1. The man + past + (Q) + (have+en) + go   The man had to have gone.

2. The boy + past + (have+en) + (Q) + go   The boy had had to go.

3. The girl + present +(Q) + (be+ing) + go   The girl has to be going.

4. Joe + present + will + (Q) + go   Joe will have to go.

In this set, let Q = *be to.*

1. Joe + present + (Q) + go   Joe is to go.

2. Fred + past + (Q) + (have+en) + (Q) + go   Fred was to have been to go.

3. The dog + past + (Q) + (be+ing) + obey   The dog was to be obeying.

In these exercises, let Q = *be about to.*

1. The baby + present + (Q) + crawl   The baby is about to crawl.

2. The building + past + (have+en) + (Q) + fall   The building had been about to fall.

3. The company + present + (Q) + (be+ing) + move   The company is about to be moving.

In these exercises, let Q = *be going to.*

1. Joe + past + shall + (Q) + go   Joe should be going to go.

2. Fred + past + (have+en) + (Q) + go   Fred had been going to go.

3. The baby + present + (Q) + (be+ing) + crawl   The baby is going to be crawling.

THE DETERMINER SYSTEM

THE DETERMINER SYSTEM of English provides the syntactic frame-work through which most numerical and quantitative information is communicated (Hargis and Ahlersmeyer, 1970; Hargis, 1971). Determiners are those words and structures which regularly occur before nouns. The noun phrase (NP) consists of a determiner (Det) plus a noun (N) or,

$$NP \longrightarrow Det + N$$

COUNT AND NONCOUNT NOUNS

Nouns can be separated into a number of classes according to certain characteristics of the things that they name. Nouns may be animate (dog, fish, boy, etc.) or inanimate (table, rock, milk, etc.). Nouns can have a variety of such characteristics or features. However, nouns can be separated into two sets in order to determine their measurable characteristics and to examine their function in relation to the determiner system. Nouns may be classed as count nouns or noncount nouns. Count nouns name things which can be counted, such as birds, toys and people. Noncount nouns name things which exist on a more continuous basis and cannot be counted. Noncount nouns include things like milk, sand, hair, etc.

Nouns and determiners constitute noun phrases. Nouns are not part of the determiner per se. However, the nature of the noun, count or noncount, exerts a selectional influence on certain determiner elements that appear before them. Also, the countability of nouns can change with context. A noun can change classes, but in any one context the noun will be either count or noncount.

THE DETERMINER

The phrase structure rule for the determiner is

Det⟶ (pre-article)^n + Article + (proximity) +
(Number)

Parenthesis indicate that those items need not be present in the determiner, but when they occur they must occur in that position in relation to the other determiner elements. Notice that *article* is the only structure that must appear in the determiner. The exponent n with the prearticle indicates that it is repeatable.

ARTICLE. The article is composed of the definite (def) article and nondefinite (nondef) articles, or

Art⟶ def, nondef

In further examination of the structure we find that the definite article consists only of *the:*

def⟶ the

Further breakdown of the nondefinite class shows it to consist of *a, an* and *some,* and Ø is called the null or zero article. The rule for nondefinite class looks like this:

nondef⟶ a(n), some, Ø

Count nouns may be preceded by all of the articles. Singular forms will be preceded by *a(n)* or *the (a* ball, *an* apple, *the* ball, *the* apple). Plural forms of count nouns may be preceded by *the, some* or the zero article *(the* balls, *some* balls, balls). Noncount nouns can be preceded by all of the same articles except a(n).

The zero article (Ø) is used to make a general statement about the class or set of things named by the noun. Count nouns preceded by Ø will be plural in form. Consider the following sentence examples with noun phrases counting the zero article as their determiner:

1. *Cars* have four wheels. (Ø cars)
2. *Apples* are often red. (Ø apple)
3. *Milk* is a liquid. (Ø milk)
4. *Hair* is primarily protein. (Ø hair)

The correct use of the definite article *(the)* is very difficult for severely hearing impaired children. However, there are a relatively few rules which govern most uses of the definite article with which these children have problems. Generally when a thing or group of things is known, it will be referred to as *the thing* or *the things:*

5. *The car* is at the corner.
6. A policeman bought *the car.*
7. *The apples* are in the refrigerator.

In examples 5, 6 and 7 the nouns in question have the sense of the specific or familiar because of the use of *the.*

If a noun is not familiar, then the first prosodic appearance of the noun will be with one of the nondefinite articles, *a(n)* or *some.* Subsequent appearances of the noun will be with *the* since it is specific and familiar due to its previous introduction:

8. John bought *a car.*
9. *The car* was a lemon.

Notice that sentence number 9 is contextually related to sentence number 8 through the definite article.

Proper nouns ordinarily do not require determiner structures. They are already sufficiently specific. However, if there is more than one person or thing with the same proper name in question, then they may be preceded by determiner structures.

PROXIMITY

The terms *demonstrative* or *demonstration* have been used in place of the term *proximity.* The term *proximity* was chosen because it seems closest to the conceptual and semantic basis of its function. Proximity is composed of *nearness* and *remoteness,* or

Proximity————→ nearness, remoteness

Proximity can only occur in the presence of the definite article *(the).* Depending on whether the following noun is singular or plural, we find that

the + nearness————→ this, these
the + remoteness ———→ that, those

Noncount nouns can be preceded only by *this* and *that* (this milk, that sand). Count nouns can be preceded by any of the four forms since they have both singular and plural forms (this car, these cars, that car, those cars).

NUMBER

The number category is composed of two subcategories which are *ordinal* and *cardinal:*

Number⟶ (ordinal) + (cardinal)

Both ordinal and cardinal numbers may appear before the noun in the noun phrase.

CARDINAL. Cardinal numbers consist of number words such as *one, two, three, four* and so on to infinity:

Cardinal⟶ One, two, three, etc.

Some noun phrase examples illustrating the sequence *cardinal +N* are *one ball, two horses, three cars.*

ORDINAL. Ordinal numbers consist of the regular ordinal number words *first, second, third, fourth, fifth* and so on to infinity. Additionally, the ordinal class contains words like *next, middle* and *last:*

Ordinal⟶ next, middle, last, first, second, third,
fourth, etc.

Ordinal numbers are usually preceded by the definite article in a noun phrase. Some noun phrase examples illustrating the sequence *def + oridinal + N* are *the first ball, the second horse, the third car.*

Notice the oneness described in all of the ordinal number noun phrases. The singular forms of nouns are used with the ordinal number alone.

Cardinal and ordinal numbers may appear together in noun phrases. In this event the structure of the noun phrase will contain first the definite article; next, the ordinal number; then the cardinal number; and, finally, the noun. Some noun phrase examples of the sequence *def + ordinal + cardinal + N* are *the first five cars, the second two trees, the last two cars.*

When ordinal and cardinal numbers appear together, the cardinal number must be greater than one. The general concept expressed by the ordinal-cardinal sequence is the ordinal position of a set. The plural form of count nouns is used with this determiner sequence.

PREARTICLES

Prearticles consist of elements such as *several of, one of, a piece of,* etc. Prearticles usually end in *of.*

The prearticles occurring with count nouns are used to refer to sets of numbers or elements of sets. They also may include cardinal numbers. Some examples of noun phrases containing these prearticles with count nouns are *one of the cars, some of the marbles, one hundred of the seeds.*

Some of the prearticles are inclusive such as *everyone of the marbles, all of the students, each of the cookies, both of the girls.*

The prearticle is the syntactic frame for fractions: consider *one half of the boys, a quarter of the girls, two thirds of the class.* These structures probably evolve conceptually from the less precise prearticles like *a piece of, a part of, some of,* etc.

The prearticle class carries the exponent n which indicates that the prearticle is repeatable as in *a piece of the slice of bread.*

Noncount nouns occurring with prearticles may or may not use the definite article: consider *a glass of the water, a glass of water, a quart of the milk, a quart of milk.*

DELETIONS. In certain instances elements of prearticles may be deleted. Some examples are *many of the boys, many boys, both of the girls, both girls.* In both of these cases the sequence *of the* was deleted.

When the noun in a noun phrase is replaced by a plural personal pronoun, the sequence looks like *several of us, some of you* or *a few of them.*

USE OF A OR AN

The choice between the nondefinite articles *a* and *an* is determined by sound, not spelling. Hearing-impaired children are more often faced with this problem. Their problem arises when words begin with a vowel, usually *u,* such as *unit or university,* but which have the consonant sound heard at the beginning of *yes* or *yesterday.*

REVIEW EXERCISES

Rewrite the following formula into noun phrase forms.

The following noun phrases contain the determiner sequence *def + proximity:*

1. def + nearness + boy   this boy
2. def + nearness + boys   these boys
3. def + remoteness + boy   that boy
4. def + remoteness + boys   those boys

Determiner consists of *prearticle + article.*

1. some of + def + boys   some of the boys
2. each of + def + boys   each of the boys
3. a lot of Ø + ice cream   a lot of ice cream

Determiner consists of *article + number.* Let ordinal = first and cardinal = five.

1. the + ordinal + boy   the first boy
2. the + cardinal + boys   the five boys
3. the + ordinal + cardinal
   + boys   the first five boys

Determiner consists of *article + proximity + number* in this set. Let ordinal = middle and cardinal = three.

1. the + nearness + ordinal
   + boy   this middle boy
2. the + remoteness +
   cardinal + boys   those three boys
3. the + nearness + ordinal
   + cardinal + boys   these middle three boys
4. the + romoteness + ordinal
   + cardinal + boys   those middle three boys

Determiner consists of *prearticle + article + proximity.*

1. a few of + def +
   nearness + boys   a few of these boys
2. each of + def +
   remoteness + boys   each of those boys

In the last set of exercises, write out the formula for the determiner in each of the noun phrases that is provided.

1. a boy	nondef + boy
2. the milk	def + milk
3. this girl	def + nearness + girl
4. one of those boys	prearticle + def + remoteness + boys
5. these four boys	def + nearness + cardinal + boys
6. that fifth girl	def + remoteness + ordinal + girl
7. each of those last four boys	prearticle + def + remoteness + ordinal + cardinal + boys
8. boys	nondef (Ø) + boys

NOUNS

NOUN FEATURES

IN THE PREVIOUS CHAPTER a feature of nouns was emphasized. This feature was countability. This feature of nouns was important in determining the form of the determiner used with them. Other noun features are important in determining which nouns can be used with certain verbs. These features are also convenient ways of classifying nouns.

CONCRETE–ABSTRACT

The noun *idea* represents a noun in the feature class which is abstract. *Rock* is a noun which is concrete. These features restrict their selection with certain verbs:

1. A *rock* fell on the car
   (but not)
*2. An *idea* fell on the car.

LIVING–NONLIVING

Nouns can be members of several feature classes. The word *rock* is a count noun, it is concrete, and it is nonliving.

3. A *carrot* is growing in the pot.
   (but not)
*4. A *rock* is growing in the flower pot.

ANIMATE–NONANIMATE

Dog is an example of a noun in the feature class of animate things. The word *carrot,* which was introduced in the class of living things, is also a member of the nonanimate class. Notice the selectional restrictions in the following examples:

    5. The *dog* coughed.
    (but not)
*6. A *carrot* coughed.

HUMAN—NONHUMAN

Boy is an example of a human noun. *Dog,* while animate, is an example of a nonhuman noun:

    7. A *boy* drew the picture.
    8. A *dog* drew the picture.

Certain verbs will utilize nouns regardless of their features. *Surprise* is such a verb:

    9. An *idea* surprised the man.
    10. A *rock* surprised the man.
    11. A *dog* surprised the man.
    12. A *carrot* surprised the man.
    13. A *boy* surprised the man.

The selectional restrictions which we have described in terms of noun features are necessary for appropriate literal interpretation of subject verb sequences. However, figurative use of language often capitalizes on violation of these restrictions. The figurative device is personification. In this example the abstract noun *courage* is in a feature position of an animate noun.

    14. *Courage* left him.

Figurative use of language will cause problems in comprehension of such structures (Hargis, 1970). Lester (1971) points out that we can make an interpretation of such relations only because we know what the correct co-occurrence relations are supposed to be.

NOUNS TO VERBS

Some quite common nouns may be changed to verbs. This change in class is a possible source of confusion to some children. Consider the following sentence pairs:

    1. The boy put the rabbit in a *cage*.
    2. The boy *caged* the rabbit.
    3. The bear is a *mother*.

4. The bear *mothered* the cubs.
5. Some *dust* is on the table.
6. Joe *dusted* the table.
7. We heard the *telehpone.*
8. They *telephoned* for help.
9. There is *air* in the room.
10. We *aired* the room.
11. We pulled a *cart.*
12. We *carted* the sludge to the garden.

VERBS TO NOUNS

The very common procedure for changing verbs to nouns is by adding the *er* suffix (if the verb ends in ate, the suffix *or* is used). This ending imparts the meaning of someone or something that does things. *Drive* becomes *driver, build* becomes *builder,* etc.

The suffix *ment* is added to verbs to make nouns. The nouns formed in this manner are abstract. *Amend* becomes *amendment; advance, advancement;* etc.

ADJECTIVES TO NOUNS

Abstract nouns may be made from some adjectives by adding the suffix *ness. Sweet* changes to *sweetness; lazy* becomes *laziness; kind* becomes *kindness;* etc.

COMPOUND NOUNS

Lees (1963) suggested a variety of ways used to produce compound nouns. These compound nouns are derived from sentences. Lees suggested some of the following derivational sources:
1. The *book* is a *text.* (textbook)
2. The *room* is *dark.* (darkroom)
3. The *lamp* is for a *table.* (table lamp)
4. The *food* is for a *dog.* (dogfood)
5. The *car* is like a *box.* (boxcar)
6. The *dog* is like a *bull.* (bulldog)
7. The *worm* cuts. (cutworm)
8. The *boat* tugs. (tugboat)

9. The man *cracks safes.* (safecracker)
10. The man *reads minds.* (mind reader)

Some of these compound nouns have a figurative basis (examples 5 and 6). These structures will pose the same problem as the simile in the base sentences from which they are derived. The last two examples (9 and 10) incorporate the *er* affixing procedure discussed earlier. Of course, many of the more common compound nouns of this type will be learned concretely without any notion of their figurative origin. Though less difficult, the other examples of compound nouns retain the meaning imparted by their different sentence bases.

PRONOUNS

PERSONAL PRONOUNS

THE PERSONAL PRONOUNS that are used in subject positions are illustrated in the following table.

Table I

SUBJECT PRONOUNS

	first person	second person	third person
singular	I	you	it, she, he
plural	we	you	they

In the first person, *I,* means the person speaking. The plural form *we* really means *I,* the speaker, plus other people. One person is acting as a spokesman for the group. It does not mean a group of speakers talking in unison.

In the second person, *you,* means the listener. There is no distinction between singular and plural forms.

Additional context is sometimes required to determine who and how many *you* and *we* represent.

1. You boys stop fighting.
2. We teachers stick together.
3. You three go to the office.

The use of first and second person pronouns is limited to the speaker-listener relationship. However, the third person pronouns are noun substitutes. The third person singular pronouns substitute for nouns on the basis of the noun's gender. *He* and *she* replace nouns simply on the basis of the known sex of the animate creature named by the noun. The nouns that *it* replaces are referred to as *neuter*. *It* automatically replaces nonanimate nouns. *It* will usually replace animate nouns when the sex is unknown.

The plural form of all third person pronouns is *they*.

The pronoun *it* has some uses which are primarily syntactic. In these instances it is very difficult to identify what *it* refers to:

3. *It* is snowing.
4. *It* is time to go.
5. *It* was me.

Personal pronouns may be used to fill various object positions in sentences. These include the indirect object of some transitive verbs and the object of prepositions. Table II illustrates the objective (or accusative) forms of personal pronouns.

Table II

OBJECT PRONOUNS

	first person	second person	third person
singular	me	you	it, her, him
plural	us	you	them

The speaker-hearer relationship is maintained through first and second person objective forms. *You* again serves both the singular and plural function in the second person objective positions.

Table III illustrates the possessive (genetive) forms of the personal pronouns.

All but one of the possessive pronouns in this table have an additional form enclosed by parenthesis. *Its,* the singular, third person, possessive pronoun cannot be used without the noun indicating the thing possessed. Consider the following sentences

Table III

POSSESSIVE PRONOUNS

	first person	second person	third person
singular	my (mine)	your (yours)	its, her (hers), his (his)
plural	our (ours)	your (yours)	their (theirs)

which show the reduction of the possessed noun:

1. The car is *my car*.   The car is *mine*.
2. *Our car* is blue.   *Ours* is blue.
3. The boy wants *your bike*.   The boy wants *yours*.
4. The boy wants *her bike*.   The boy wants *hers*.
5. *His bike* has ten gears.   *His* has ten gears.
6. *Their corn* is flourishing.   *Theirs* is flourishing.
7. The dog wants *its food*.
      (but not)   *The dog wants *its*.
8. The bone is *its bone*.
      (but not)   *The bone is *its*.

In most cases the possessed noun may be deleted if some available context makes it easily known. In sentence 1 the possessed noun is supplied in the subject position. It is not only known, it is redundant and is most often deleted in these circumstances. However, these conditions do not permit the reduction of the possessed noun following *its* (sentences 7 and 8).

Many of the (so-called) errors which occur in using personal pronouns have to do with confusing subject and object placement of pronouns:

*1. He sat between Helen and I.
*2. Fred and me are going.
*3. Me and him had fun.

The bulk of these *errors* occur when a conjunction is used to join a noun or pronoun to another pronoun.

NOUN REDUCTION

Nouns are often deleted from noun phrases when there is sufficient context and when a noun is repeated in the sentence:

1. *This car* is my car.	*This* is my car.
2. *These mittens* are mine.	*These* are mine.
3. *That ball* is mine.	*That* is mine.
4. I want *those apples*.	I want *those*.
5. *One apple* fell from the table.	*One* fell from the table.
6. *That one apple* has a worm in it.	*That* one has a worm in it.

In examples 1 through 4 the noun is omitted from the noun phrase, leaving the determiner element to supply any additional context that is needed to make identification of the missing noun possible. All of these could be reduced to personal pronouns.

These reduced forms pose a number of conceptual and syntactic problems for children. One problem is the reduction of information which will then require extra use of context. Another is the problem of *clozure* across the syntactic gaps which are left by the reduction processes.

REFLEXIVE PRONOUNS

If an object of a sentence is the same as the subject, then a reflexive pronoun will be used in the object position. They are formed by adding *self* to pronoun forms. Reflexive pronouns are illustrated in Table IV.

Table IV

REFLEXIVE PRONOUNS

	first person	second person	third person
singular	myself	yourself	himself, itself, herself
plural	ourselves	yourselves	themselves

The object positions include object of a preposition as well as direct and indirect objects:

1. Joe bought a suit by himself.
2. It hurt itself.
3. We bought ourselves a new car.

The reflexive pronouns may also be used to intensify (Thomas, 1965; Streng, 1972) :

4. Joe *himself* drank the last beer.
5. Joe drank the last beer *himself*.
6. I *myself* heard it.
7. I heard it *myself*.

Notice that when a reflexive is used to intensify a sentence it may move from the position following its referent noun to the end of the sentence. Refer to sentences 5 and 7.

INDEFINITE PRONOUNS

Indefinite pronouns are a group of twelve, which are composed in the manner illustrated in the following table:

Table V

INDEFINITE PRONOUNS

	body	one	thing
every	everybody	everyone	everything
some	somebody	someone	something
no	nobody	no one	nothing
any	anybody	anyone	anything

Only *no one* is written as two words. Even though the term *indefinite* implies indefiniteness in meaning, those formed with *every* and *no* seem rather definite. There is a possible source of confusion with these pronouns. Even when those that seem plural are used as subjects of sentences, they require the singular form of whatever verb is used:

1. Everybody goes.　　　(but not)　*Everybody go.
2. Everyone is happy.　　(but not)　*Everyone are happy.
3. Everything runs fine. (but not)　*Everything run fine.

Some children may have difficulty separating the meaning and the use of those indefinite pronouns beginning with *some* and *any*.

When a sentence is negative or contains certain negative structures, the indefinite pronouns beginning with *some* are generally not used:

4. The boy didn't like anything.
5. The child seldom eats anything.
6. Joe didn't ask everybody.

The indefinite pronouns formed by *no* may be used in place of those formed by *any* in the verb phrase of negative sentences:

7. The boy didn't like anything. The boy liked nothing.
8. Joe doesn't have anything.　　Joe has nothing.

However, there is no equivalence of the *no* and *any* forms if the indefinite pronouns are in the subject position of negative sentences.

9. Anything doesn't please
   the boy.　　　　　　　(is not)　Nothing pleases the boy.
10. Anything can't
    happen.　　　　　　　(is not)　Nothing can happen.

Some children may have difficulty in separating the meaning and use of those indefinite pronouns beginning with *some* and *any*. The following examples are intended to illustrate some differences:

11. I will bet on anything.
12. I will bet on something.

In example 11 *anything* refers to any member of the set of things which might be bet on. In example 12 *something* refers to only one unspecified member of the set of things which can be bet on. *Some* indefinites seem to refer to only one unspecified member of a set, and *any* indefinites refer to each of the members of the set without specification.

THE NEGATIVE TRANSFORMATION

THE NEGATIVE TRANSFORMATION

THE NEGATIVE in English is varied in function. The negative will be reconsidered in some of the subsequent chapters and illustrated as a function of the structures and transformations introduced therein. Several kinds of negation are functions of the auxiliary, and this type of negation will receive the most attention here. One corollary topic, *affirmation,* will be considered.

NEGATION IN THE AUXILIARY

In Chapter 3 a rule for the auxiliary was introduced.

Aux ———→ Tense + (Modal) + (have+en) + (be+ing)

The negative's appearance in the auxiliary varies systematically according to what appears in the auxiliary of a sentence. The following illustrations and examples will deal with negation as it occurs with each auxiliary element. If tense alone appears in the auxiliary of a sentence, then the appearance of the negative will be determined by the sentence's verb. The negative particle (not) is introduced by means of the negative transformation (T-neg).

TENSE AND BE. If *be* is the verb and only tense occurs in the auxiliary of the same sentence, then the T-neg will insert *not* immediately following *be.*

　　　1. NP + present + be + adj　　　The girl is happy.
T-neg

　　　NP + present + be + not
　　　+ adj　　　　　　　　　　　　The girl is not happy.
　　　2. NP + past + be + NP　　　　The car was a Ford.

T-neg

NP + past + be + not

+ NP   The car was not a Ford.

Most of the verb forms of *be,* including *is, are, was* and *were,* form contractions in the negative. These are, respectively, *isn't, aren't, wasn't* and *weren't.*

TENSE AND OTHER VERBS

All verbs other than *be* require an additional element to form the negative when they have only tense in their auxiliaries. This element is *do. Do* is inserted transformationally (T-do) between *tense* and *not.* Consider these examples, illustrating first the *positive* form of the sentence, then T-neg and then T-do:

3. NP + past + VT + NP   The boy made cake.

T-neg

NP + past + not + VT + NP

T-do

NP + past + do + not +   The boy did not make

VT + NP   cake.

Notice that no actual sentence is possible until after *T-do* is applied. Tense cannot affix to the negative particle. It is necessary to insert *do* in order to provide a holder for tense.

4. NP + present + VT + NP   The boy makes cake.

T-neg

NP + present + not + VT

+ NP

T-do

NP + present + do + not   The boy does not make

+ VT + NP   cake.

Notice in example 4 that *do* will carry the affix indicating subject and verb agreement. Present tense singular is *does.* Present tense plural is *do,* so, in addition to providing a holder for tense, *do* is also a holder for plural-singular indicators in the present tense. The next examples illustrate the application of *T-neg* to sentences with verbs in the *have* and intransitive classes:

5. NP + present + have + NP   The girls have a dog.

T-neg

> NP + present + not +
> have + NP

T-do

NP + present + do + not + have + NP	The girls do not have a dog.
6. NP + present + VI	The bird flies.

T-neg

NP + present + not + VI	
NP + present + do + not + VI	The bird does not fly.

The negative will form contractions with the inserted *do. Do, does* and *did* are respectively *don't, doesn't* and *didn't*.

To summarize, when tense is the only element occurring in the auxiliary, the negative transformation will make required the *do* transformation with verbs other than *be. Do* will carry the indicators of tense and number after the negative transformation. The negative transformation inserts *not* after *be* when it is the verb with only tense in its auxiliary.

OTHER AUXILIARY ELEMENTS. When more elements than just tense occur in the auxiliary of a sentence, the negative particle will normally be inserted after the element which follows tense. The *do* insertion will no longer be required. These conditions are true whether or not *be* or other verbs are used in the sentence. The first set of examples illustrates the negative transformation of sentences which contain the auxiliary sequence tense + (modal):

7. NP + present + will + be + adj	The girl will be happy.

T-neg

NP + present + will + not + be + adj	The girl will not be happy.
8. NP + present + can + have + NP	The girl can have a dog.

T-neg

NP + present + can + not + have + NP	The girl cannot have a dog.
9. NP + present + must + go	The children must go.

T-neg

NP + present + must   The children must not
+ not + go   go.

Some of the modals with negative particles will form contractions. *Can, will, shall, must* and *need* become *can't, won't,
shan't, mustn't* and *needn't* in the present tense. The modal *need*
requires a negative, either with it or with a noun or noun phrase
in the sentence in which it occurs:

10. The boy need not come.
11. No boy need come.

The past tense forms of the modals *could, would* and *should*
also form contractions. Respectively, they are *couldn't, wouldn't*
and *shouldn't*.

The following examples illustrate the result of the negative
transformation on sentences containing the auxiliary sequence
tense + (have+en) :

12. NP + present +
    (have+en) + go   The boy has gone.

T-neg

NP + present + have
+ not + en + go   The boy has not gone.

13. NP + past + (have+en)
    + be + adj   The boy had been good.

T-neg

NP + past + have + not   The boy had not been
+ en + be + adj   good.

Notice that *not* is inserted after *have* in the auxiliary element
(*have+en*). The negative particle will form the contractions
haven't, hasn't and *hadn't*.

In the next set of examples the negative transformation is performed on sentences containing the auxiliary sequence tense +
(be+ing) :

14. NP + present + (be+ing)
    + run   The girl is running.

T-neg

    NP + present + be + not

    + ing + run   The girl is not running.

15. NP + past + (be+ing)   The boy was driving a

    + VT + NP   car.

T-neg

    NP + past + be + not   The boy was not driving

    + ing + VT + NP   a car.

Not is inserted after *be* in the auxiliary element (*be+ing*). The negative particle will form the same contractions with the auxiliary *be* that it did with the verb *be*.

If the next element after *tense* in the auxiliary of a sentence is a quasi-modal, the second word in the auxiliary will be either *have* or *be*. When the Q is *have to,* then *do* insertion is required.

16. NP + past + (have to)

    + go   Fred had to go.

T-neg

    NP + past + not +

    (have to) + go

T-do

    NP + past + do + not   Fred did not have to go.

    + (have to) + go

17. NP + present + (have to)

    + be + adj.   He has to be good.

T-neg

    NP + present + not +

    (have to) + be + adj

T-do

    NP + present + do + not   He doesn't have to be

    + (have to) + be + adj   good.

Examples 16 and 17 show that the negative is formed with the sequence *tense* + (*have to*) in the same way that the negative is formed with the sequence *tense* + *have* when *have* is the verb of the sentence.

All of the other quasi-modals begin with *be*. When a quasi-modal which begins with *be* is the first element after tense in the auxiliary, then the negative is formed in the same way as all other sequences of *tense* + be ... form the negative.

18. NP + present + (be going
      to) + go   He is going to go.

T-neg

      NP + present + be + not
      + going to + go   He is not going to go.

19. NP + present + (be about
      to) + fly   The bird is about to fly.

T-neg

      NP + present + be + not
      + about to + fly   The bird is not about to
                                    fly.

20. NP + present + (be
      unable to) + work   He is unable to work.

T-neg

      NP + present + be + not
      + unable to + work   He is not unable to
                                    work.

The net result in this last example is, however, a positive rather than negative interpretation.

AFFIRMATION

The negative transformation inserted the negative particle *not* in various auxiliary positions or following the verb *be*. When the sequence tense plus any verb other than *be* or the Q *have to* occurred, then *do* insertion was required.

The affirmative transformation (T-affirm) operates in much the same way as the negative. The main difference being that instead of the negative particle, the particles *so* or *too* are inserted. The effect of this transformation is to affirm the information provided by the sentence. The transformation will not make a sentence positive. It only affirms the sentence's statement.

The following examples show the affirmative transformation on sentences containing some of the auxiliary elements and verb classes:

1. NP + present + have + NP   Joe has a dog.

T-affirm

NP + present + $\binom{so}{too}$ +
have + NP

T-do

NP + present + do +

$\binom{so}{too}$ + NP   Joe does $\binom{so}{too}$ have a dog.

2. NP + present + be + NP   She is a teacher.

T-affirm

NP + present + be +

$\binom{so}{too}$ + NP   She is $\binom{so}{too}$ a teacher.

3. NP + past + VT + NP   She hit the boy.

T-affirm

NP + past $\binom{so}{too}$ + VT
+ NP

T-do

NP + past + do $\binom{so}{too}$ +   She did $\binom{so}{too}$ hit the boy.
VT + NP

4. NP + present + will + VI   She will run.

T-affirm

NP + present + will

$\binom{so}{too}$ + VI   She will $\binom{so}{too}$ run.

5. NP + present + (be+ing)
+ VI   She is running.

T-affirm

NP + present + be +

$\binom{so}{too}$ + ing + VI   She is $\binom{so}{too}$ running.

6. NP + present + (have+en)
+ VI   She has run.

T-affirm

NP + present + have +

$\binom{so}{too}$ + en + VI   She has $\binom{so}{too}$ run.

The affirmative transformation may be performed on a
sentence without the insertion of *so* or *too*. In this case, whichever

word would normally be followed by *so* or *too* would, instead, receive stress. Stress means that the word would be spoken with more than normal intensity. The *do* insertion is still a requirement with the sequence's tense plus verbs other than *be* or the Q (*have to*). The italicized words in the following examples receive stress:

7. Joe *does* have a dog.
8. She *is* a teacher.
9. She *did* hit the boy.
10. She *will* run.
11. She *is* running.
12. She *has* run.

THE NEGATIVE WITH NOUN PHRASES

The negative particle *no* appears to function in a noun phrase in any position which can be occupied by the nondefinite articles *a(n), some, Ø*. If this form of negation is used, it seems to be essentially synonymous with auxiliary negation in the same sentence:

1. No boy was in the barn. (=) A boy was not in the barn.
2. They had no shoes. (=) They didn't have shoes.

The negative particle *not* appears to function in prenoun phrase positions rather than within the noun phrase as *no* does:

3. *Not a boy* was in the room.
4. *Not any of the students* came.
5. *Not one of students* came.
6. *None of the students* came.
7. *Not much of the candy* was left.
8. *Not many of the children* came.
9. *Not all of the candy* was gone.

Examples 4, 5 and 6 are essentially synonymous. *Not any of, not one of* and *none of* appear to produce the same meaning. There are a number of restrictions on the use of *any of*. One condition under which it can be used is—if it is preceded by the negative particle. Consider the following unacceptable example:

*10. Any of the students came.

The prearticles *some of* and *each of* generally are not preceded by not.*
  *11. Not some of the candy was good.
  *12. Not each of the boys had toys.

The definite article will generally not be preceded by the negative particle.†
  *13. Not the boy came.

Acceptable forms of 11, 12 and 13 are formed with the negative in the auxiliary:
  14. Some of the candy was not good.
  15. Each of the boys did not have toys.
  16. The boy did not come.

More attention to the negative will be necessary in association with other syntactic areas. The most complete work which has been done on negation is by Edward S. Klima (1964). Students who are interested in an intact consideration of this subject are well referred to it.

---

*This can happen under certain conditions which are discussed in connection with conjunctions.

†This occurrence is also possible in connection with certain conjunctions.

PREPOSITIONAL PHRASES

A LICE STRENG (1972) LISTS sixty simple prepositions and twenty-five compound prepositions which she feels represent those in common use in English today. Of this group of prepositions, only nine *(at, by, for, from, in, of, on, to* and *with)* account for about 90 percent of the actual occurrences of prepositions (Fries, 1940). These are relatively few, but the average number of meanings for each of the nine prepositions is thirty-six and a half. This multiplicity of meaning poses one of the significant problems the language-impaired child has in mastering structures containing prepositions.

We have discussed one prepositional form, the *of* used with prearticles. We will consider or reconsider some of these prepositions in subsequent chapters on phrasal verbs, indirect objects, possessives, nominalizing transformations, the passive transformation and adverbials. These various usages pose the second significant problem in mastery of these structures.

The prepositions under consideration in this chapter are restricted to those in prepositional phrases. These phrases are composed of a preposition(s) plus a noun phrase or nominal.

TIME PHRASES

The prepositions that frequently function in time phrases are listed below:

about	before	during	near	to	until
after	between	from	on	through	within
around	beyond	in	since	throughout	
at	by	inside	till	up to	

Most of these prepositions cannot by themselves be linked with time. They all require a noun or nominal form which conveys a time meaning in order to function as time phrases. Of this list of prepositions only *during, since, till* and *until* are restricted to time functions.

The very common prepositions, *at, in* and *on,* frequently function in time phrases. These take forms such as *at noon, in the morning, at nine o'clock* and *on Tuesday.* The problems which occur expressively with these time phrases usually have to do with interchanging their uses inappropriately. *At* is used to indicate specified times during the day as in *at lunch, at three o'clock,* etc. *On* is used with days of the week or specified days as in *on Tuesday, on Christmas Day,* etc. *In* is used with months, seasons and years. Some examples are *in June, in the winter* and *in 1963.*

There is some common use of the three prepositions in time phrases, but each of the three areas just illustrated is more exclusively the domain of a particular one of them.

The prepositional phrases used as adverbials of time have considerably more freedom of movement than do other prepositional phrase forms. From the following examples, you can see that the time phrase can move to either end of the sentence which it modifies.

1. I go to work *on Monday* (or) *On Monday* I go to work.
2. Fred always has a party *on his birthday* (or) *On his birthday,* Fred always has a party.

Time phrases may occur with any sentence type. The other prepositional phrases are more limited in their usage, and many have functions determined by the verb phrase of the sentence type in which they appear.

PHRASES FOLLOWING BE

In the chapter on sentence classes, two prepositional phrase forms were introduced in sentences which had the verb *be.* These were called the adverb of purpose and the adverb of place. Examples of these are as follows:

3. The gift is *for you.*

4. The bird is *in a tree.*
5. Fred is *at work.*

Prepositional phrases like these which function as a part of the verb phrase are often called *complements.*

One additional prepositional phrase needs to be considered with *be* class sentences. When *be* is followed by an adjective, on certain occasions this adjective can be followed by a prepositional phrase.

1. Joe is *afraid of the dog.*
2. Zeke is *happy for Helen.*
3. Pete was *amazed at the trick.*
4. He is *ashamed of his clothes.*
5. They are *sensitive to criticism.*
6. Joe is *conscious of his appearance.*

Notice that the adjectives used in the sequence *be + adjective + prepositional phrase* describe states that are mental or emotional.

PHRASES FOLLOWING INTRANSITIVE VERBS

Some sentences with intransitive verbs require adverbial complements. This verb group was discussed briefly in Chapter 2. It contains verbs like *hang, stand, live, glance,* etc. This complement position is readily filled by place phrases:

1. The picture hangs *on the wall.*
2. The boy stood *in the corner.*
3. She lived *in New York.*
4. He glanced *at her.*

Some prepositional phrases express more motion than place. When a prepositional phrase expresses motion, the noun phrase part of the phrase is deletable:

1. Joe walked *out of the store.*
   Joe walked *out.*
2. Helen drove *through the city.*
   Helen drove *through.*
3. The dog ran *into the room.*
   The dog ran *in.*

4. They walked *up to the second floor.*
   They walked *up.*
5. They walked *over to the park.*
   They walked *over.*

Notice that if two prepositions are used, the second one is dropped. This includes the *to* from *into.* The reduction of information in this way permits efficiency of expression, but it requires the effective use of context to *cloze* over the missing elements.

PHRASES FOLLOWING NOUNS IN THE VERB PHRASE

In Chapter 2 we mentioned one transitive verb which required adverbials of place in the position following its direct object noun phrase:

1. He put the pot *on the stove.*
2. They put their money *in the bank.*

These prepositional phrases appear to be more like adverbs of motion. Notice that the prepositions could be expanded to *on to* and *into,* respectively. Also, the noun phrases following these prepositions may be deleted.

Other transitive verbs may be followed by adverbs of motion as well.

3. She drove the cab *into the lot.*
   She drove the cab *in.*
4. He lifted the box *up to the shelf.*
   He lifted the box *up.*
5. They pushed the car *up the hill.*
   They pushed the car *up.*

There are a variety of other prepositional phrase types which occur following noun phrases used as objects.

6. They made the statue *of clay.*
7. They made the house *from brick.*
8. They built the house *with logs.*
9. They filled the box *with sand.*
10. They thanked Fred *for the present.*
11. They left the car *in the garage.*
12. They returned the gift *to the store.*

13. They changed the nightclub *into a garage*.
14. They took pity *on him*.

Obviously the prepositions in these examples are varied in meaning and in usage. *Of, from* and *with* in examples 6, 7 and 8 have roughly the same meaning. However, they may be used in entirely divergent ways.

INDIRECT OBJECTS

The prepositions *for* and *to* are used to introduce the indirect objects when they follow transitive verbs. The following sentences contain examples of these phrase forms of prepositional phrases:

15. Joe gave the cigarettes *to Fred*.
16. Helen brought the candy *for Betty*.
17. Joe paid the dollar *to the store*.

Under certain conditions the indirect object can be moved and the prepositions deleted. This will be discussed in more detail in the chapter on indirect objects.

POSSESSIVES

Two prepositions, *of* and *with,* are used to indicate possession. Exampes with *of* are

1. The handle *of the broom* broke. (the broom's handle)
2. The cover *of the book* is red. (the book's cover)
3. The brother *of Joe* came. (Joe's brother)

Though possession is also indicated by *with,* the meaning is not equally synonymous to the possession indicated by *of:*

4. The door *with the brass knob* is open.
5. Joe bought a shirt *with long sleeves*.

BY PHRASES

The preposition *by* will frequently perform in place phrases as in

1. Fred sat *by Mary*.
2. The shoe was *by the bed*.

They can be used in adverbs of motion and their noun phrase may be deleted:

3. Joe drove *by the house.*   Joe drove *by.*
4. The postman comes *by the*   The postman comes *by* at
house at noon.   noon.

By can be used in phrases that indicate means or manner:
5. He came *by boat.*
6. They traveled *by camel.*

Passive sentences constitute one of the more difficult forms in which *by* will appear:
7. The tree was struck *by lightning.*
8. The car was washed *by Fred.*

The agent subject of the sentence is the noun phrase following *by* in these sentences. The problem here may be partly due to the difficulty children have with passive sentences as well as the multiple use of *by.*

MULTIPLE PREPOSITIONS

Jespersen (1933) suggested that prepositional phrases themselves could be the object of prepositions:
1. from *behind the tree*
2. from *over the bridge*
3. since *before the war*
4. persons of *from sixteen to twenty-six*

These examples, however, may be no different from other complex prepositions in use, some of which have been mentioned with adverb or motion phrases. Other common sequences are *back to, up from, from over, across from,* etc. However, some compound prepositions appear in indefinite units such as *in front of, in back of, in spite of, on account of,* etc.

MULTIPLE PREPOSITIONAL PHRASES

Some prepositional phrases seem to go naturally in pairs:
1. The boys walked *from school to the store.*
2. The boys were on vacation *from June until August.* Multiple prepositional phrases of time are readily used:
3. The boys left *at noon on Monday*

Multiple adverbs of place may be used until the number becomes stylistically unacceptable or until the speaker-hearer's performance limitation precludes further comprehension.

4. There is a bug on the leaf of a tree by the house.

Prepositional phrases indicating possession may be linked indefinitely but with the same limitations expressed above.

5. Joe saw the car of the cop of the police force of Jonesboro.

Aside from time, place, purpose, possession and agent, which have been briefly discussed, other uses of prepositional phrases include manner, means, concomitance, reason and likely other uses. These may appear in sentences in various combinations as needed.

6. He bought the bike for Jerry for Christmas at the hardware store.

Except for the indirect objects (for Jerry) the sequence of occurrence for the other prepositional phrases seems optional.

NEGATIVE USES

One phrase is used quite frequently as a tag on sentences which are negative. This phrase is *at all*.

1. I don't want that *at all*.
2. He had no money *at all*.

This phrase is idiomatic and seems to be used to emphasize the negative aspect of the sentence.

One preposition, *with,* can form a negative. The negative form is *without:*

3. Joe didn't come *with* Fred.
4. Joe came *without* Fred.

VARIOUS USES OF PREPOSITIONS

It was mentioned earlier that prepositions had multiple meanings. Some of these meanings must occur because of the multiple functions which they serve. Consider the following examples of *with:*

1. Joe played *with Fred*.
2. Joe hit Fred *with a board*.
3. Joe bought a car *with four doors*.

4. He is *with the group.*
5. He bowed *with a flourish.*
6. He died *with pneumonia.*
7. Joe played *with the blocks.*

In sentences 1 through 6, the phrase indicates accompaniment, instrument, possession, place, manner and reason, respectively. The total sentence context must provide some restrictions which help select or narrow down the meaning for *with* in each of its different functions. This use of context is necessary for dealing with all of the more common prepositions.

The last usage (sentence 7) is an example of a prepositional verb which will be discussed in the next chapter. Many of the prepositions which are under consideration for their function in prepositional phrases will also occur as parts of verbs as well as parts of prepositional phrases. This other common function further compounds the difficulty of mastering prepositional phrases.

PHRASAL VERBS

NEW VERBS CAN BE MADE in English by adding prepositions to existing verbs. The terms used to describe these verbs include double verb, two-word verb, prepositional verb, verb particle and phrasal verb. The author's selection of *phrasal verb* is arbitrary.

Verb formation in this manner is quite common in English:

1. He *dropped out.*
2. They had to *clean up* the mess.
3. They *broke out* of jail.
4. Someone *held up* the bank.
5. The pitcher *psyched out* the batter.
6. You can *count on* Fred.
7. He *let in* the guest.
8. She *ran across* an old friend.

There are several problems in coping with phrasal verbs. These are dealing with a preposition or particle as a part of the verb and separating the use of prepositions with the verb and with a preposition phrase. Since very often the phrasal verb is figurative or idiomatic, a problem occurs when trying to identify the literal meaning through a figurative device.

Concerning the last problem, a sentence might be interpreted two ways, depending upon whether the preposition is part of the verb or a part of a prepositional phrase:

9. They *decided on* the farm.
10. They decided *on the farm.*
11. He *ran across* a strange bird.
12. He ran *across a strange bird.*

In sentence 9 the phrasal verb *decided on* indicates that the farm was chosen or selected. However, in sentence 10 *on* is the preposition heading the prepositional phrase *on the farm,* which indicates where some decision was made. Notice also that *decided on* is a transitive verb while *decided* in sentence 10 is intransitive.

The next examples show the idiomatic as well as the relatively literal and concrete use of the same phrasal verb:

13. The suspenders *held up* his trousers.
14. The robber *held up* the bank.

The literal interpretation of the idiomatic and figurative phrasal verbs is a persisting problem. Many new phrasal verbs enter the language often as slang or through current events.

15. Someone *ripped off* my bike.
16. The pitcher *psyched out* the batter.
17. The music *turned on* the audience.
18. A number of medical instruments have *spun off* from space technology.
19. Civil rights workers *sat in* at the Bijou.

Many phrasal verbs also nominalize readily, so we can find some of our previous examples appearing as some of the following nouns

20. This is *a rip-off*.
21. There was *a hold-up* at the bank.
22. He is *a drop-out*.
23. *A run-away* was picked up by the sheriff.
24. *A spin-off* of the meeting was a date with Elsie.

Phrasal verbs enrich the language, but they are always a potential source of confusion to anyone having a problem learning English.

INTRANSITIVE PHRASAL VERBS

Phrasal verbs can be intransitive:

1. The papers *stacked up*.
2. The money *ran out*.
3. He *gave in*.
4. They *held out*.

5. He will *turn up*.
6. The watch *ran down*.
7. He *struck out*.
8. They *hurried on*.
9. I *woke up*.

Mark Lester (1971) suggests that even the verb *be* can be used as an intransitive verb if it has an affixed preposition. He provides these examples:

10. The batter *is up*.
11. The batter *is out*.
12. The game *is over*.

TRANSITIVE PHRASAL VERBS

The following set of examples contains transitive phrasal verbs:

1. Fred *scuffed up* his shoes.
2. He *picked out* a new tie.
3. The conservatives *took over* the parliament.
4. He *stacked up* the dishes.
5. Ali *knocked out* his opponent.
6. He *made up* a story.
7. He *put on* his coat.

Many of the prepositions can be shifted from the position next to the verb to the position following the object noun phrase. This shifting of the preposition is a *transformational* rule which applies to the moveable prepositions in transitive phrased verbs. This shifting transformation is applied to the phrasal verbs in the following sentences, resulting in the equivalent transformed sentences:

8. Fred *pulled up* his socks. (becomes) Fred *pulled* his socks *up*.
9. He *took back* the tie. (becomes) He *took* the tie *back*
10. They *took over* the ownership. (becomes) They *took* the ownership *over*.
11. He *stacked up* the boxes. (becomes) He *stacked* the boxes *up*.

12. Joe *passed out*
    cigars.   (becomes) Joe *passed* cigars *out.*
13. He *made up* a
    story.   (becomes) He *made* a story *up.*
14. She *put on* the
    record.   (becomes) She *put* the record *on.*

Whenever the object noun phrase is a personal pronoun, the shifting transformation becomes mandatory:

*15. Fred *pulled up*   (must
     them.   become) Fred *pulled* them *up.*
*16. He *took back* it.   (must   He *took* it *back.*
                            become)

The shifting transformation is optional if the object noun phrase is not a personal pronoun.

The shift of the preposition in some phrasal verbs is not possible. Some of them have inseparable prepositions. These verbs behave as if they were single-word verb units.

17. We *rely on* her.   (but   *We *rely* her *on.*
                           not)
18. They shot at the   (but
    rabbit.   not)   *They *shot* the rabbit *at.*
19. They checked into   (but   *They *checked* the story
    the story.   not)   *into.*

Inseparable phrasal verbs include *run across, hear of, depend on, look into, look after, cope with, confide in, get around, stand by, learn about, get over,* etc.

Though not a transitive verb, *have* will form a phrasal verb with the preposition *on.* The result, *have on,* is replaceable by the verb *wear.* The preposition *on* will also shift.

1. She *had on* a coat.   (or)   She *had* a coat *on.*
2. Joe *has on* his   (or)   Joe *has* his pajamas *on.*
   pajamas.

CONCLUSION

Phrasal verbs pose a good many varied problems to the language handicapped child. They are often figurative, and these may be confused with preposition phrase structures. Some intransitive verbs form phrasal verbs, but phrasal verb formation is quite common in transitive verbs. In the case of separable phrasal verbs, the prepositional particle may shift to either side of object noun phrases. When the object noun phrase is a personal pronoun, then the particle must be shifted to the position following the personal pronoun. Some phrasal verbs are inseparable. The particle cannot be separated from the primary verb.

In addition to the functions and the problems illustrated above, rather complex-looking sequences of prepositions may appear as the result of the appearance of phrasal verbs with prepositional phrases in some of the forms mentioned in the last chapter:

1. They walked *on by* (us) .
2. The dog crawled *back in under* (the house) .
3. Bring *on over* your friend. (and even)
4. Come *on back over* to my house.

Bolinger (1971) , among others, treats the subject of phrasal verbs extensively. Makkai (1972) considers these phrasal verbs which function idiomatically. The readers interested in further study of phrasal verbs are recommended to these works.

EXERCISES

Shift the particles in the following sentences:

1. The boy *picked up*   The boy *picked* the ball
   the ball.   *up*.
2. The lady *let in* the cat.   The lady *let* the cat *in*.
3. Dad *woke up* the dog.   Dad *woke* the dog *up*.

In the following sentences, change the object noun phrases to personal pronouns and then shift the particles, if possible.

4. The hotel *put up*   The hotel *put* them *up*.
   the scouts.
5. We *depend* on Fred.   We *depend on* him.
                                  (no shift)
6. The dog *knocked down*   The dog *knocked* him *down*.
   the boy.
7. They *can cope with* the   They can *cope with* it.
   inflation.   (no shift)
8. She *put away* the paper.   She *put* it *away*.

CHAPTER 11

INDIRECT OBJECTS

SOME TRANSITIVE VERBS will take indirect objects. Several examples of these were presented in the chapter on prepositional phrases. The prepositions *to* and *for* are the fundamental ones which are used to introduce the phrase forms of indirect objects. The indirect object will appear in its phrase form following the object noun phrase:

1. They bought the present *for father.*
2. They sent some flowers *to Jill.*
3. They gave some candy *to April.*
4. They found a place *for Linda.*

All of the indirect objects listed in examples above can undergo a transformational change that moves the indirect object from the position following the object noun phrase to the position before it. When this movement occurs, the preposition is deleted:

5. They bought the present *for father.*	(becomes)	They bought *father* the present.
6. They sent some flowers *to Jill.*	(becomes)	They sent *Jill* some flowers.
7. They gave some candy *to April.*	(becomes)	They gave *April* some candy.
8. They found a place *for Linda.*	(becomes)	They found *Linda* a place.

There is one restriction on the indirect object shift transformation. This restriction occurs when the object noun phrase is a personal pronoun. When this happens, then the indirect object will appear in the phrase form only:

9. They brought it *for father.*	(but not)	*They brought *father* it.

10. They sent them *to Jill.*	(but not)	*They sent *Jill* them.
11. They gave it *to April.*	(but not)	*They gave *April* it.
12. They found it *for Linda.*	(but not)	*They found *Linda* it.

Care must be taken to distinguish *for* phrases which are not indirect objects from those which are:

13. We bought the soap *for Fred.*
14. She sent the package *for Joe.*

Sentences 13 and 14 are ambiguous because the prepositional phrase in each may be interpreted as either an indirect object or as a prepositional phrase of the type described in Chapter 9. This second interpretation is one of *assistance.* In sentence 13 the prepositional phrase *for Fred* could mean that the soap was purchased at Fred's request to assist him. In sentence 14 the phrase *for Joe* could mean that the package was sent to Joe (the indirect object) or that the package was sent to assist Joe at his request, quite likely to some other person. This is a fairly narrow range where confusion of this sort can develop. No confusion is possible if the indirect object shift transformation is performed when this is the intended meaning. Consider the following sentences which show the result of the indirect object shift transformation on sentences 13 and 14:

15. We bought *Fred* the soap.
16. We sent *Joe* the package.

If, on the other hand, the nonindirect object meaning is intended, then some additional contextual information would be necessary to correctly interpret the sentence.

Some transitive verbs such as *see, hear, let, want, surprise* and *please* do not have indirect objects:

17. April surprised Jill for Fred.
18. Linda pleased the teacher for mother.

Notice that in both of these examples the indirect object interpretation is not possible. Also notice that since the *for* phrases are not indirect objects, the indirect object shift transformation cannot apply. Consider the following grammatically incorrect results of this transformation applied to sentences 17 and 18:

*19. April surprised *Fred* Jill.

*20. Linda pleased *mother* the teacher.

EXERCISES

If possible, put the following sentences through the indirect object shift transformation:

1. The boy will give the bone to the dog.

    The boy will give the dog the bone.

2. The class bought it for the teacher.

    (not applicable)

3. The mother gave the toy to her son.

    The mother gave her son the toy.

4. Father will take ice cream to his son.

    Father will take his son ice cream.

CHAPTER 12

YES/NO QUESTIONS

Some questions require either a yes or a no answer. These questions constitute the class of questions which are the topic of this chapter. They take forms such as

1. Do you like strawberry ice cream?
2. Is that dog a poodle?
3. Will you come to the party?
4. Have they eaten lunch?
5. Does Fred have a dog?

There is only one circumstance where questions formulated in this way won't require a *yes* or *no* response. This occurs when the question contains the conjunction *or:*

6. Do you like strawberry *or* chocolate ice cream?
7. Is that dog a poodle *or* a great dane?
8. Will you come to the party *or* go to the game?
9. Have they eaten lunch *or* breakfast?
10. Does Fred have a dog *or* a cat?

In these examples, the question requires that a choice be made between the alternatives presented. The answer, rather than a simple *yes* or *no,* will be one of the alternatives.

AUXILIARY AND VERB MOVEMENT

As in the negative transformation, the *yes* and *no* question transformation (T-yes/no) is dependent on the structure of the auxiliary or the type of verb contained in the transformed sentence. When tense alone occurs in the auxiliary, then the type of verb will determine the form of the question.

Tense and Be. If only tense occurs with the verb *be,* then the question transformation will shift the sequence *tense + be* to the front of the sentence:

    1. NP + present + be +

T-yes/no

      adj   The girl is happy.

    2. NP + past + be +

T-yes/no

      NP   Is the girl happy?

Tense and Other Verbs. The verbs other than *be* generally require an additional transformation when they have only tense in their auxiliaries. This transformation is the insertion of *do* (T-do). In sentences such as these, T-yes/no will shift only *tense* to the front of the sentence while the verbs other than *be* will remain in their original position in the sentence. After *tense* is shifted, then T-do is required to carry the original indicators of tense as well as subject and verb agreement. Consider these examples.

    3. NP + past + VT + NP   The boy made cake.

T-yes/no

      past + NP + VT + NP

T-do

      past + do + NP + VT

      + NP   Did the boy make cake?

    4. NP + present + VT + NP   The boy makes cake.

T-yes/no

      present + NP + VT + NP

T-do

      present + do + NP + VT

      + NP   Does the boy make cake?

Notice that no actual sentence is possible without the insertion of *do.*

The next examples illustrate the application of T-yes/no to sentences containing the sequence *tense + have:*

    5. NP + present + have + NP   The girls have a dog.

T-yes/no

      present + NP + have + NP

T-do

    present + do + NP + have

    + NP   Do the girls have a dog?

    6. NP + past + have + NP   The children had fun.

T-yes/no

    past + NP + have + NP

T-do

    past + do + NP + have   Did the children have

    + NP   fun?

Also possible, but much less common, is the shift of the sequence *tense + have* to the front of the sentence:

    7. NP + present + have + NP   Joe has a car.

T-yes/no

    present + have + NP + NP   Has Joe a car?

In this example, no *do* insertion is required since *have* is available to carry indicators of tense and agreement.

With intransitive verbs, the transformational sequence is the same as for transitive verbs.

    8. NP + present + VI   The bird flies.

T-yes/no

    present + NP + BI

T-do

    present + do + NP + VI   Does the bird fly?

    9. NP + past + VI   The boy ran.

T-yes/no

    past + NP + VI

T-do

    past + do + NP + VI   Did the boy run?

OTHER AUXILIARY ELEMENTS. When elements in addition to tense occur in the auxiliary of a sentence, T-yes/no will shift tense plus the first word which follows it to the front of the sentence. First, consider the examples which contain the auxiliary sequence *tense + (Modal):*

    10. NP + present + will

    + adj.   The girl will be happy.

T-yes/no
> present + will + NP
> + be + adj.   Will the girl be happy?

11. NP + present + can
> + have + NP   The girl can have a dog.

T-yes/no
> present + can + NP
> + have + NP   Can the girl have a dog?

12. NP + past + shall + go   The children should go.

T-yes/no
> past + shall + NP + go   Should the children go?

The next examples illustrate the results of the *yes* and *no* question transformation on sentences containing the sequence *tense + (have+en):*

13. NP + present + (have+en)
> + go   The boy has gone.

T-yes/no
> present + have + NP
> + en + go   Has the boy gone?

14. NP + past + (have+en)
> + be + adj   The boy has been good.

T-yes/no
> past + have + NP + en
> + be + adj   Had the boy been good?

Notice that the auxiliary element (have+en) is divided by T-yes/no. *Have* moves with tense to the front of the sentence and *en* remains in its original position.

In the following examples T-yes/no is performed on sentences containing the sequence *tense + (be+ing):*

15. NP + present + (be+ing)
> + run   The girl is running.

T-yes/no
> present + be + NP +
> ing + run   Is the girl running?

16. NP + past + (be+ing)   The boy was driving a
> + VT + NP   car.

T-yes/no

past + be + NP + ing + VT + NP	Was the boy driving a car?

In examples 15 and 16 the auxiliary element (be+ing) is divided by T-yes/no. *Be* moves with tense to the front of the sentence and *ing* remains in its original position.

If the next element in the auxiliary after tense is a quasi-modal, the second word in the auxiliary will be either *have* or *be*. When the *Q* is *have to*, then tense alone will shift to the front of the sentence and *do* insertion is required. When the *Q* begins with *be*, then *tense* plus *be* will shift to the front of the sentence:

17. NP + past + (have to)
   + go   Fred had to go.

T-yes/no

   past + NP + (have to)
   + go

T-do

   past + do + NP + (have
   to) + go   Did Fred have to go?

18. NP + present + (be going
   to) + be + adj   He is going to be good.

T-yes/no

   present + be + NP +
   going + to + be + adj   Is he going to be good?

If the sentence being transformed contains a negative, then the negative particle will move to the front of the sentence along with the other appropriate structures.

19. NP + past + do + not
   + VI   He did not go.

T-yes/no

   past + do + not + NP
   + VI   Didn't he go?

20. NP + present + will
   + not + VI   He will not go.

T-yes/no

   present + will + not
   + NP + VI   Won't he go?

The graphic representation of these question forms includes the question mark at the end of the sentence. In speech the last word in yes/no questions has a higher pitch level.

ECHO QUESTIONS

Yes/no questions may be formulated without auxiliary or verb movement. A sentence can be transformed into a yes/no *echo* question by changing the pitch contour of any nonquestion sentence to that appropriate to the regular yes/no questions where the last word in the sentence is produced at a higher pitch level. Clear representation of these questions is only possible in speech. Graphically, the only clue that these sentences are questions is the placement of a question mark at the end of the sentence. Questions formed in this manner carry a note of incredulity or surprise.

TAG QUESTIONS

Apparently, the most difficult of the yes/no question forms is the "tag" question (Brown and Hanlon, 1970). Again, the formulation of these yes/no questions is a function of the auxiliary or the verb class. In addition, however, the form that these questions takes is influenced by whether or not the sentence is negative:

1. Joe went, *didn't he?*
2. The girl will buy the car, *won't she?*
3. The dog has run home, *hasn't it?*
4. Mother is making a cake, *isn't she?*

Notice that in each of these examples a sentence is made a question by adding a *tag* to the base sentence. The tags for sentences 1 through 4 are respectively *didn't he, won't she, hasn't it* and *isn't she.* Notice also that if the base sentence contains no negative, then the tag must. The negative will usually appear in a contracted form. However, more formal expression of the tags with negatives leaves the negative particle at the end of the tag as in *will she not, has it not* or *is she not.*

Consider the following examples where the base sentences do

contain a negative:

5. Joe did *not* go, *did he?*
6. The girl will *not* buy a car, *will she?*
7. The dog has *not* run home, *has it?*
8. Mother is *not* making a cake, *is she?*

Notice that if the base sentence is negative, then the tags will not contain a negative.

Other components of this question transformation include repetition of tense and the first element in the auxiliary which follows it at the end of the sentence, then the pronoun form of the base sentence's subject is added at the end of the tag. As indicated in examples 1 and 5, the *do* insertion is used when only tense occurs in the auxiliary together with verb forms other than *be*.

EXERCISES

Transform each of the following sentences into (1) regular yes/no questions, (2) echo questions and (3) tag questions:

1. The doctor was sick.

Was the doctor sick?
The doctor was sick? (echo)
The doctor was sick, wasn't he?

2. The children played.

Did the children play?
The children played? (echo)
The children played, didn't they?

3. Father had been building the house.

Had father been building the house?
Father had been building the house? (echo)
Father had been building the house, hadn't he?

4. They will have to come.

Will they have to come?
They will have to come? (echo)
They will have to come, won't they?

5. The nurse does not have   Doesn't the nurse have to work
   to work today.   today?
                              The nurse does not have to
                                work today? (echo)
                              The nurse does not have to
                                work today, does she?

CHAPTER 13

WH QUESTIONS

WE HAVE DISCUSSED the first major type of questions in the last chapter. Those questions can be answered by *yes* or *no*. This chapter presents questions which ask for particular pieces of information. They are called *wh* questions because most of them begin with interrogative words that start with the letters *wh*. The interrogative words which begin them include *who, whom, whose, which, what, where, when, why, how, how often, how much* and *how many*. Consider the following *wh* questions with their corresponding answers:

1. Where does Joe live?   Joe lives at *the beach.*
2. When is your birthday?   My birthday is *May 30.*
3. What can you bring?   I can bring the *dessert.*
4. Who lives at the beach?   *Joe* lives at the beach.
5. How many pets do you have?   I have *three* pets.

The questions are directed to the italicized elements. This short italicized element alone would be quite acceptable as the answer to the questions.

The various question words have a relationship to the type of element they are eliciting. *What* is used for nonanimate noun phrases, *who* with human and some animate noun phrases, *where* with adverbs of place, *how many* with number, *why* with adverbs of reason or cause, etc.

Wh questions like the yes/no questions are transformations of other sentences. Additionally, *wh* questions share a number of characteristics with yes/no questions. Specifically, we find the same auxiliary and verb movement in both question types. The same application for *do* insertion occurs in both as well. The *wh* question transformation incorporates the features of the yes/no question transformation but additionally replaces some sentence structures with an interrogative word.

WH QUESTION TRANSFORMATION

It was pointed out that the *wh* question transformation (T-wh) incorporates the structural features of T-yes/no in addition to the replacement of certain sentence structures by appropriate interrogative words:

1. Joe wanted a car.
2. Did Joe want a car? (by T-yes/no)
3. What did Joe want? (by T-wh)
4. Who wanted a car? (by T-wh)

Examples 2, 3 and 4 are transforms of a sentence like number 1. To view these sentences transformationally we can break the auxiliary into its constituent parts and observe each of the question transformations which follow.

5. NP + past + VT + NP   Joe wanted a car.

T-yes/no

past + NP + VT + NP

T-do

past + do + NP + VT
+ NP   Did Joe want a car?

6. NP + past + VT + NP   Joe wanted a car.

T-yes/no

past + NP + VT + NP

T-wh

what + past + NP + VT

T-do

what + past + do + NP   What did Joe want?
+ VT

Notice that the first step in producing this *wh* question was to move *tense* by T-yes/no. Then, by applying T-wh, the NP which is *a car* is replaced by the appropriate interrogative word and moved to the front of the sentence. After T-wh is applied, then *do* insertion is necessary to carry tense. This last step will produce the *wh* question, *what did Joe want?*

7. NP + past + VT + NP   Joe wanted a car.

T-yes/no

past + NP + VT + NP

T-wh

who + past + VT + NP   Who wanted a car?

In example 4 the *wh* question, *Who wanted a car?* is produced by first applying T-yes/no and then T-wh.

Notice that no *do* insertion is required in this example. This can occur when a subject noun phrase is replaced by *who* or *what* and moved to the front. This movement again leaves tense next to the main verb.

Basically, *wh* questions follow the format, first T-yes/no and then T-wh. If necessary then *do* insertion will be last. The one exception with T-do was illustrated in example 4.

The *wh* questions have a different intonation pattern from yes/no questions. Yes/no questions have higher intonation on the last word while *wh* questions have the falling intonation of simple sentences.

T-WH, NOUN PHRASE

The type of interrogative word used in *wh* questions depends upon the word or structure which it is to replace transformationally. This interrogative word is also a primary clue as to the nature of the specific answer the question is eliciting. The interrogative words *who, whom* and *what* are used to replace noun phrases. *Who* will be used with human subject noun phrases. *Who* is commonly used to replace noun phrases which are direct objects, indirect objects and objects of prepositions. However, the more literary form uses *whom*. *What* is used for most nonhuman and nonanimate nouns:

1. NP + present + will +
   VT + NP   *Mary* will help *Fred.*

T-yes/no

present + will + NP +
VT + NP

T-wh

    who + present + will +

    VT + NP   Who will help Fred?

T-wh replaced the subject NP with *who* and shifted to the front of the structure produced by T-yes/no. Replacing the direct object, which is Fred in example 1, we can get this question by T-wh.

T-wh

    Who(m) + present + will

    + NP + VT   Who(m) will Fred help?

The next example shows the replacement of all three noun phrases by the three possible T-wh noun phrase transformations.

    2. NP + present + (be+ing)   *Mary* is buying *the candy*

    + VT + NP + for + NP   for *Fred.*

T-yes/no

    present + be + NP + ing

    + VT + NP + for + NP

T-wh

    Who + present + be + ing   Who is buying the candy

    + VT + NP + for + NP   for Fred?

               [or]

T-wh

    What + present + be + NP   What is Mary buying for

    + ing + VT + for + NP   Fred?

               [or]

T-wh

    Who(m) + present + be +

    NP + ing + VT + NP   Who(m) is Mary buying

    + for   the candy for?

In the last question transformation there is some objection to ending sentences with prepositions. In this case it is the preposition *for* which introduces an indirect object. In more formal expressions, the sequence *preposition + noun phrase* may be shifted by T-wh when the noun phrase being replaced is the object of a preposition. Consider the more formal form of this *wh* question:

    3. *For whom* is Mary buying the candy?

Any of the other prepositions may shift with the interrogative words *who(m)* or *what:*

4. NP + present + VT + NP   He put the money in *the*
   + in + NP   *bank.*

T-yes/no

present + NP + VT + NP
+ in + NP

T-wh

What + past + NP + VT
+ NP + in

T-do

what + past + do + NP   What did he put the
+ VT + NP + in   money in?
          [or]

T-wh

in + what + past + NP
+ VT + NP

T-do

in + what + past + do   In what did he put the
+ NP + VT + NP   money?

DETERMINER INTERROGATION. Determiners or portions of determiners, which with nouns constitute noun phrases, can be subject to interrogation just as can the entire noun phrase. The interrogative words which are used to replace determiner structures are *which, how many* and *how much.*

5. NP + past + buy + def
   + remoteness + N   Joe bought *that* car.

T-yes/no

past + NP + buy + def
+ remoteness + N

T-wh

which + N + past + NP
+ buy

T-do

which + N + past + do
+ NP + buy   Which car did Joe buy?

Notice that the determiner element is replaced by the word *which* and then the entire noun phrase, including *which,* is shifted to the beginning of the sentence. *How many* is used to interrogate certain determiner structures used with count nouns. Again the appropriate determiner element is replaced and the whole noun phrase is shifted to the beginning of the sentence:

6. *A few* of the apples		How many of the apples
	(becomes)	
were wormy.		were wormy?
7. *Six boys* left		How many boys left
	(becomes)	
early.		early?

How much is used to interrogate some determiner elements which occur before noncount nouns:

8. *A quart* of milk		How much of the milk
	(becomes)	
was frozen.		was frozen?

WHOSE. The interrogative word *whose* is used to replace possessive animate or human nouns and pronouns. You may notice that *whose* replaces the appropriate possessive form and moves together with the noun which follows to the beginning of the sentence.

9. Joe bought *Fred's*		Whose car did Joe buy?
	(becomes)	
car.		

10. *Joe's* car is red.   (becomes) Whose car is red?

This question form will be considered in further detail in the chapter on possessives.

With question forms *which, how many, how much* and *whose,* the noun which is shifted with the question word may be deleted when context is sufficient. Questions would then be like

11. Which did Joe buy?
12. How many were wormy?

T-WH, ADVERBIAL

In situations where various adverbial structures are to be interrogated, the appropriate interrogative words must be selected. *Where* replaces adverbs of place; *when* replaces adverbs of time; *how* replaces adverbs of manner and instruments, among others; *how often* replaces adverbs of frequency, and so on.

1. Joe *carefully* put   How did Joe put out the
   (becomes)
   out the fire.   fire?

2. Joe put out the   Where did Joe put out
   (becomes)
   fire *at school*.   the fire?

3. Joe put out the   How did Joe put out the
   (becomes)
   fire *with some water*   fire?

4. Joe put out the   When did Joe put out
   (becomes)
   fire *yesterday*.   the fire?

How was used to interrogate two different adverbial constructions (examples 1 and 3). *How* is used with a large number of different structures; many are adverbial but many are not. *How* is used as a simple interrogative word and in compounds such as *how often, how many, how much, how come, how far* and *how long*. It is likely for these reasons that *how* questions pose some of the greatest difficulty for children.

The *why* question form is another particularly difficult question form. *Why* is not used with the wide number of structures that *how* is, but it is used to interrogate some conceptually and syntactically complex forms (Hargis, 1975). Basically, *why* replaces adverbial structures of cause or reason.

5. They took the horses to   Why did they take the
   (becomes)
   the river *for them to*   horses to the river?
   drink.

A wide variety of structures can indicate cause or reason. These structures as well as the *why* question forms will be considered in detail in the chapter on cause and effect.

Two other interrogative elements are essentially synonymous with *why*. These are *how come* and *what――for*. Consider the following example where all three questions are derived from the same sentence:

6. The girls like vacations	Why do the girls like
(becomes)	
because they go to the	vacations?
beach.	(or)
	How come the girls like
	vacations?
	(or)
	What do the girls like
	vacations for?

Notice that in the *how come* form there is no yes/no component. In all *how come* questions the interrogative element simply replaces the causal or reason structure and moves to the beginning of the sentence.

SPECIAL PROBLEMS

One common construction can be the source of some confusion. This occurs when the adjective which follows sense verbs is interrogated. *How* is used to replace this adjective. This seems to be the only circumstance when an adjective is replaced by an interrogative word.

1. NP + present + VS + adj   The candy tastes *sour*.

T-yes/no

present + NP + VS + adj

T-wh

How + Present + NP + VS

T-do

How + present + do + NP + VS	How does the candy taste?
2. NP + present + will + VS + adj	The water will feel *warm*.

T-yes/no

present + will + NP + VS + adj

T-wh

How + present + will +	How will the water
NP + VS	feel?

The confusion with this form may result from the more frequent adverbial or determiner replacements with *how*.

Another question form which poses even greater problems uses the interrogative words *what kind of*. Also similar are *what type of, what brand of, what make of,* etc. This question form is directed to various kinds of noun modifier words or structures.

3. He bought a *Ford*	What kind of tractor did
(becomes)	
tractor.	he buy?
4. He wears *an old*	What kind of hat does he
(becomes)	
wornout hat.	wear?

The difficulty of this question form is likely due to the level of complexity of the noun modifier which it is interrogating.

Another question form which is extremely difficult for many language handicapped children is *what happened?* Forms of this question may be directed to a specific structure in sentences or to the sentence as a whole. Consider these two questions from sentence 5.

5. The boy fell.	(becomes)	What happened?
		[or]
		What happened to the boy?

This question, however, is frequently directed to whole sequences of events and the answer requires a recounting of the events or a summary of them.

    6. What happened yesterday?

    7. What happened on your vacation?

    8. What happened when you were in the army?

The ability to comprehend and answer these questions requires mastery of ordering sequence of events, the ability to summarize and all the necessary sentence forms to accurately relate the component occurrences.

WH QUESTIONS WITHOUT T-YES/NO

This *wh* question is formed by replacing the interrogated element by the proper *wh* question word. The question word is not shifted. This *wh* question word is then given emphasis or stress in the question:

1. John gave Fred *the*   John gave Fred what?
   (becomes)
   ball.

2. John gave *Fred* the   John gave who the ball?
   (becomes)
   ball.

3. *John* gave Fred the   Who gave Fred the ball?
   (becomes)
   ball.

In example 3 you may notice that the derived question could result from T-yes/no and a regular T-wh question transformation.

It is even possible to interrogate more than one element in one sentence using this device:

4. Fred hit *Joe*   Fred hit who(m) when?
   (becomes)
   yesterday.

It is also possible to use both forms of *wh* questions to interrogate more than one sentence component:

5. Why did he go where?
6. What did who want?

Quigley, Wilbur and Montanelli (1974) studied question formation in the language of deaf children from ages ten to nineteen. Their study points out the general difficulty which profoundly prelingually deaf children have in comprehending and in judging the grammaticality of question forms. This study also pointed out the same order of difficulty and age of emergence for deaf as for normal children, which was noted in studies by Brown and Hanlon (1970). The major stages of development of question forms were the same, although deaf students go through them much later in their chronological development.

EXERCISES

Perform all of the necessary transformations to arrive at the appropriate *wh* questions. The questions are to be directed to the italicized elements in each of the following sentences:

1. The lady bought *a hat.*

   The lady + past + buy + a hat

   T-yes/no

   past + the lady + buy + a hat

   T-wh

   what + past + the lady + buy

   T-do

   what + past + do + the lady + buy
   What did the lady buy?

2. *The girl* will be a doctor.

   the girl + present + will + be + a doctor

   T-yes/no

   present + will + the girl + be + a doctor

   T-wh

   who + present + will + be + a doctor
   Who will be a doctor?

3. The dog ran in *the yard.*

   the dog + past + run + in + the yard

   T-yes/no

   past + the dog + run + in the yard

   T-wh

   where + past + the dog + run

   T-do

   where + past + do + the dog + run
   Where did the dog run?

4. The baby is
hugging *the toy*.

    the baby + present + (be
+ing) + hug + the toy

T-yes/no

    present + be + the baby
+ ing + hug + the toy

T-wh

    what + present + be +
the baby + ing + hug

5. The floor feels
cold.

    What is the baby hugging?
the floor + present + feel
+ cold

T-yes/no

    present + the floor + feel
+ cold

T-wh

    how + present + the floor
+ feel

T-do

    how + present + do + the
floor + feel
How does the floor feel?

6. The dog chased
the man.

    the dog + past + chase +
the man

T-yes/no

    past + the dog + chase +
the man

T-wh

    who(m) + past + the dog
+ chase

T-do

    who(m) + past + do + the
dog + chase
Who(m) did the dog chase?

7. The boy has to go
by bus.

    the boy + present + (have
to) + go + by bus

T-yes/no

present + the boy + (have to) + go + by bus

T-wh

how + present + the boy + (have to) + go

T-do

how + present + do + the boy + (have to) + go
How does the boy have to go?

8. *Four* students were sick.

four students + past + be + sick

T-yes/no

past + be + four students + sick

T-wh

how many students + past + be + sick
How many students were sick?

9. They drank a *quart of* milk.

they + past + drink + a quart + of milk

T-yes/no

past + they + drink + a quart of milk

T-wh

how much milk + past + they + drink

T-do

how much milk + past + do + they + drink
How much milk did they drink?

10. He caught a fish *with his hand.*

he + past + catch + a fish + with his hand

T-yes/no

> past + he + catch + a fish
> with his hand

T-wh

> how + past + he + catch
> + a fish

T-do

> how + past + do + he +
> catch + a fish
> **How did he catch a fish?**

CHAPTER 14

WHAT—DO QUESTIONS

━━━━━━━━━━━━━━━━━━━━━━━━━━━━━━

T HE QUESTION FORM under consideration in this chapter was separated from the other *wh* question forms because it is used to interrogate the verb phrase of some sentence types. It can be produced from sentences containing intransitive and transitive verbs. It is not used freely with most copulative verb forms.

Consider these examples of transitive and intransitive sentences and their *what—do* question forms:

    1. Joe *wrecked his*   What did Joe do?
                   (becomes)
     car.
    2. Helen will *run.*   (becomes) What will Helen do?

These question forms are of frequent use and superficially appear quite simple. Notice, however, that in example 1 there is only one word, *Joe,* remaining from the sentence from which it was derived. *Do* has replaced the entire verb phrase in both examples 1 and 2. In example 1 this replacement includes an object noun phrase. Also, the interrogative word *what* is used in these question forms. This is the source of confusion with some children as they expect *what* to be the clue for a nonhuman or nonanimate noun.

Do is an abstract replacement for the verb phrase. It acts as a verbal *proform* which together with the interrogative word *what* is to elicit a verb phrase answer. Another problem with this question form is the double appearance of *do* when there is only tense in the auxiliary of the sentence.

The following examples show how the *what—do* question is formed when only tense occurs in the auxiliary:

3. NP + present + run   The dog *runs.*

T-yes/no

present + NP + run

T-wh-do

what + present + NP + do

T-do

what + present + do
+ NP + do   What does the boy do?

4. NP + past + throw + NP   The girl *threw the ball.*

T-yes/no

past + NP + throw + NP

T-wh-do

what + past + NP + do

T-do

what + past + do + NP
+ do   What did the girl do?

The first step in producing the *what—do* questions is performing T-yes/no. Next, T-wh-do is performed by replacing the verb phrase with *do* and *what,* then shifting *what* to the beginning of the sentence. In examples 3 and 4 *do* insertion is required to carry tense.

The next example shows how sentences containing the auxiliary sequence *tense + (have+en)* are transformed by T-wh-do:

5. NP + past + (have+en)   Joe had *broken the win-*
+ VT + NP   *dow.*

T-yes/no

past + have + NP + en
+ VT + NP

T-wh-do

what + past + have + NP
+ do   What had Joe done?

Notice that in example 5 *en* affixes to *do* to form the participial *done. Do* will carry any auxiliary affix which was carried by the verb that is being interrogated.

The next example shows the transformation of a sentence containing the auxiliary sequence *tense + (be+ing):*

6. NP + present + (be+ing)
   + VI   Mary is *running*.
T-yes/no

present + be + NP + ing
+ VI

T-wh-do

what + present + be + NP
+ ing + do   What is Mary doing?

Again *do* accepts the auxiliary affix which was carried by the interrogated verb. In example 6 the affix is *ing*.

With quasi-modals the transformation looks like—

7. NP + present + (Q) + VI   Joe *has to go*.

T-yes/no

present + NP (Q) + VI

T-wh-do

what + present + NP +
(Q) + do

T-do

what + present + do + NP   What does Joe have to
+ (Q) + do   do?

It is possible to form *what—do* questions without the T-yes/no component and without shifting *what*. In this example *what* is left with *do* in the original verb phrase position:

8. The boy will rake   The boy will do what?
                (becomes)
   the leaves.

As with the other *wh* questions formed without T-yes/no and without the interrogative word shift, the interrogative word requires stress or emphasis in speech.

One additional variation of this question form may be used with object noun phrases:

9. Joe hit Fred.   (becomes) What did Joe do to Fred?
10. Fred broke the   What did Fred do to the
                (becomes)
    clock.   clock?

In these examples the object noun phrase is retained. The

preposition *to* is used to introduce the object in the question form.

The apparent simplicity or the seeming resemblance to other *wh* question forms masks the syntactic complexity of these question forms. They deserve more careful systematic consideration in language curricula.

EXERCISES

Perform the necessary transformations to produce the appropriate *what—do* question from the given sentences.

1. The lady can buy the farm.

the lady + present + can + buy + the farm

T-yes/no

present + can + the lady + buy + the farm

T-wh-do

what + present + can + the lady + do

What can the lady do?

2. The baby crawls.

the baby + present + crawl

T-yes/no

present + the baby + crawl

T-wh-do

what + present + the baby + do

T-do

what + present + do + the baby + do

What does the baby do?

3. The girl had been playing ball.

the girl + past + (have+ en) + (be+ing) + play + ball

T-yes/no

past + have + the girl + en + (be+ing) + play + ball

T-wh-do

what + past + have + the
girl + en + (be+ing) +
do
**What had the girl been do-
ing?**

4. Fish have to swim　　　　fish + present + (have to)
   in water.　　　　　　　　+ swim + in water

T-yes/no

present + fish + (have to)
+ swim + in water

T-wh-do

what + present + fish +
(have to) + do

T-do

what + present + do +
fish + (have to) + do
What do fish have to do?

TRANSITIVE VERB COMPLEMENTS

I N THE CHAPTER on sentence classes the basic nature of sentences containing transitive verbs was presented. The chapters on phrasal verbs and indirect objects described two more elaborations of this same sentence class:

1. Fred threw the ball.
2. Zeke stacked the boxes up.
3. Joe gave the ball to Fred.

Sentence 1 is the simplest form. Sentence 2 contains the phrasal verb, and sentence 3 has an indirect object (to Fred) in addition to the direct object (the ball).

The structures which are a part of the verb phrase, in addition to the verb itself, are often called verb phrase complements. The complements which will be considered in this chapter are of a complex nature. These complements are sentences that are embedded in the position following some transitive verbs.

INFINITIVE PHRASES

When the complement formed by embedding a sentence takes the form of an infinitive phrase, the *tense* of the embedded sentence is replaced by the infiinitive marker *to*. When the subject of the embedded sentence is the same as the main sentence, then the subject of the embedded sentence is omitted. The italicized portion indicates the embedded sentence complement.

1. Joe wants *to eat candy*.
2. April likes *to play games*.

The embedded sentences in examples 1 and 2 are these sentences, respectively:

3. Joe eats candy.
4. April plays games.

These complex sentences are produced by a transformation which permits certain transitive verbs to embed sentences as infinitive phrases in the subject or complement position. This transformation may be called T-VT$_{to}$. In the next example this transformation is represented by embedding a sentence in the complement position following the transitive verb. The complement position is the blank following the transitive verb, and the sentence to be embedded is shown below it. The sentence resulting from T-VT$_{to}$ is shown to the right:

1. I tried _____.

T-VT_{to} (results in) I tried *to ride a mule.*

I rode a mule.

Notice that the subject is deleted from the embedded sentence and that tense is replaced by the infinitive marker *to*.

If the subject of the embedded sentence is different than the subject of the main sentence, then it will be retained as in

2. I want _____.

T-VT_{to} I want *Fred to play baseball.*

Fred plays baseball.

Verbs like *begin, hope, continue, pretend,* etc., require that the subject of the embedded sentence be the same as the main sentence. Others permit the subject to be either different or the same. Verbs such as *ask, tell, urge, force,* etc., require that the subject of the embedded sentence be different. With this latter group of verbs the subject can be the same, but it must be changed to a reflexive pronoun by the embedding transformation:

3. Fred told *himself to study hard.*
4. Joe forced *himself to get up.*

In other situations where the embedded sentence has a different subject, which is a pronoun, then the pronoun will be changed to its objective form:

5. Helen likes ——————.

*T-VT*_{*to*}   Helen likes *her to play the piano.*

She plays the piano.

The regular modal form will not embed in these infinitive phrases. We cannot have sentences like

*6. He likes *to can run fast.*
*7. He wanted *to will go.*

Occasionally congenitally deaf children will make errors such as these, indicating they have not learned this particular restriction.

Quasi-modals are not restricted as are the regular modals from being embedded through T-VT_{to}. Consider these examples where quasi-modals have been substituted for the regular modals in examples 6 and 7:

8. He likes *to be able to run fast.*
9. He wanted *to be going to go.*

Aside from tense and the regular modals, all other auxiliary elements can be retained in the embedded sentences:

10. Joe wanted *Fred to be swimming with him.*
11. Fred wanted *to have gone with Joe.*

One subset of transitive verbs, which will embed sentences as infinitive complements, will not use the infinitive marker *to.* This set of verbs includes *let, help, see, hear, watch,* etc. The transformation which embeds infinitive phrases following these verbs will be called T-VT_(to).

This set of verbs requires a different subject in the embedded sentence or the use of a reflexive pronoun if the subset is the same.

12. Joe saw ——————.

*T-VT*_{*(to)*}   Joe saw *Fred come.*

Fred came.

13. Helen helped ——————.

*T-VT*_{*(to)*}   Helen helped *Fred change the tire.*

Fred changed the tire.

Notice that tense is erased in the embedded sentence, but the resultant sentence does not contain the infinitive marker before the embedded verb.

PARTICIPIAL PHRASES

When the complement formed by embedding a sentence takes the form of a participial phrase, the *tense* of the embedded sentence is replaced by *ing*.

1. He found *Joe eating an apple*.
2. He started *running*.

This transformation is very similar to T-VT$_{to}$. The only apparent syntactic difference is the replacement of tense with *ing*. In the next example the embedding of a sentence as a participial phrase in the complement position following certain transitive verbs will be illustrated. This transformation will be called T-VT$_{ing}$.

3. They enjoyed _____.

T-VT$_{ing}$ They enjoyed *going* to
                                                 the beach.
They went to the beach.

A number of the transitive main verbs can embed sentences as either infinitive or participial phrases. These verbs include *begin, continue, start, like, try, attempt,* etc.

4. Joe tried *to shoot baskets*.
5. Joe tried *shooting baskets*.
6. Fred liked *to go to the movies*.
7. Fred liked *going to the movies*.

Other verbs, however, require the use of *ing*. These verbs include *miss, enjoy, consider, practice,* etc.

8. Joe missed *going to the beach*.
9. They enjoyed *swimming in the ocean*.

Verbs like *hear, see, watch* and *let,* which embed sentences without the infinitive marker *to,* can also embed sentences as participial phrases:

10. Joe heard *Fred snore*.
11. Joe heard *Fred snoring*.

When the main sentence contains transitive verbs like *see*, *hear* or *feel*, the participial phrase form will be used to indicate that whatever was seen, heard or felt continued for a period longer than the actual observation.

The greatest problem which children will have in using the appropriate phrase form for the complement will be when the verbs are fairly close semantically but have restrictions on which phrase forms can be used with them. Two such verbs are *enjoy* and *like*. *Like* may be followed by either an infinitive or a participial phrase while *enjoy* can be followed only by the participial forms.

BE DELETION COMPLEMENTS

The last transitive verb class to be discussed is one which permits only sentences which contain the verb *be* to be embedded as complements. When a sentence is embedded as a complement of one of these transitive verbs, both *tense* and the *be* verb are deleted. This transformation will be called T-VT$_{(be)}$. Transitive verbs which permit this embedding transformation include *keep*, *make*, *elect*, *regard*, *think*, etc. Some examples of this transformation are

1. We elected _____.

T-$VT_{(be)}$ (results in)   We elected *John president.*

John is president.

2. The fire keeps _____.

T-$VT_{(be)}$ The fire keeps *us warm.*

We are warm.

3. Sugar makes _____.

T-$VT_{(be)}$ Sugar makes *the tea sweet.*

The tea is sweet.

The embedded sentence in these transformations must have a different subject than the main sentence.

Some verbs such as *regard* permit the word *as* to be inserted where *tense* and *be* have been deleted:

4. We regard *the statement as untrue.*

QUESTION FORMS

The complements embedded by $T\text{-}VT_{to}$, $T\text{-}VT_{(to)}$ and $T\text{-}VT_{ing}$ can be the focus of interrogation in the *wh* question transformation. Normally the interrogative word *what* will replace the entire infinitive or participial phrase:

1. Mother wants Fred to   What does mother want?
   (becomes)
   eat lunch.

2. Joe found Fred   What did Joe find?
   (becomes)

It is also possible to interrogate the verb phrase of the sentence which has been embedded by the same transformations. The question form is a slight modification of the *what—do* question form.

3. Mother wants Fred   What does mother want
   (becomes)
   to eat lunch.   Fred to do?

4. Joe found Fred   What did Joe find Fred
   (becomes)
   smoking in bed.   doing?

Notice that *do* replaces the verb of the embedded sentence. The infinitive marker *to* will precede *do* or the *ing* will affix itself to *do* in infinitive or participial phrases respectively.

MULTIPLE OCCURRENCES

Sentence complexity can be increased considerably by multiple embeddings. Sentences may be embedded by one of the transitive verb transformations which already has an infinitive or participial complement. Consider the following sentences and the sequence of embedding transformations which they contain:

1. We like to watch   We like _____.
   $$T\text{-}VT_{to}$$
   the birds flying.   We watch _____.
   $$T\text{-}VT_{ing}$$
   The birds fly.

2. Mother made the   Mother made _____.
$$T\text{-}VT_{to}$$
children try to cut   The children tried
the grass.   _____.
$$T\text{-}VT_{to}$$
The children cut the
grass.

The sentences produced by the transitive verb complement transformations may be short and are quite common, but they pose a complex set of language learning problems. Each of their restrictions and forms may need to be considered carefully and introduced systematically.

EXERCISES

Identify the base sentences (main and embedded sentences) for the following sentences. Also identify whether $T\text{-}VT_{to}$, $T\text{-}VT_{(to)}$, $T\text{-}VT_{ing}$ or $T\text{-}VT_{(be)}$ produced each sentence.

1. Father let the boy   Father let _____.
   ride the horse.
   $$T\text{-}VT_{(to)}$$
   The boy rode the horse.

2. The teacher is making   The teacher is making
   the students write on   _____.
   the board.
   $$T\text{-}VT_{(to)}$$
   The students write on
   the board.

3. The nurse needed to be   The nurse needed
   going to the hospital.   _____.
   $$T\text{-}VT_{to}$$
   The nurse was going to
   the hospital.

4. The children watched   The children watched
   themselves dance.   _____.

$$T\text{-}VT_{(to)}$$

They danced.

5. The children had heard   The children had heard
   the glass break.   _____.

$$T\text{-}VT_{(to)}$$

The glass broke.

6. The girl wanted to   The girl wanted
   have eaten some candy.   _____.

$$T\text{-}VT_{to}$$

The girl has eaten some
candy.

7. Father is permitting   Father is permitting
   Mary to take a trip.   _____.

$$T\text{-}VT_{to}$$

Mary takes a trip.

8. The police would have   The police would have
   forced the students to   forced _____.
   sit down.

$$T\text{-}VT_{to}$$

The students sat down.

9. A girl saw the boys   A girl saw _____.
   fighting.

$$T\text{-}VT_{ing}$$

The boys fought.

10. I like to hear people   I like _____.
    laughing.

$$T\text{-}VT_{to}$$

I hear _____.

$$T\text{-}VT_{ing}$$

People laugh.

11. The man kept watering   The man kept
    the plants.   _____.

$$T\text{-}VT_{ing}$$

The man watered the
plants.

12. Mother had heard the   Mother had heard
    baby crying.   _____.

$$T\text{-}VT_{ing}$$

	The baby cried.
13. The class considers Tom a clown.	The class considers _____.

$$T\text{-}VT_{(be)}$$

	Tom is a clown.
14. The raincoat is keeping my clothes dry.	The raincoat is keeping _____.

$$T\text{-}VT_{(be)}$$

	My clothes are dry.
15. The man will believe the idea absurd.	The man will believe _____.

$$T\text{-}VT_{(be)}$$

	The idea is absurd.
16. Mom thinks him a fool.	Mom thinks _____.

$$T\text{-}VT_{(be)}$$

	He is a fool.
17. The students had to elect Zeke president.	The students had to elect _____.

$$T\text{-}VT_{(be)}$$

	Zeke is president.
18. The man regards his son a genius.	The man regards _____.

$$T\text{-}VT_{(be)}$$

	His son is a genius.
19. The pepper will make the food hot.	The pepper will make _____.

$$T\text{-}VT_{(be)}$$

	The food is hot.
20. The fire left the family destitute.	The fire left _____.

$$T\text{-}VT_{(be)}$$

The family is destitute.

THE PASSIVE TRANSFORMATION

T HE PASSIVE TRANSFORMATION applies to sentences which have transitive verbs. This transformation shifts the object to the subject position, and *be* plus the participle affix *en* are inserted in the auxiliary before the transitive verb. The original subject may be optionally retained at the end of the sentence following the preposition *by:*

    1. Joe broke the bat.   The bat was broken by

               (becomes)

                       Joe.

Symbolically, the passive transformation for example 1 may be illustrated in this way:

    2. NP_1 + past + break

       + NP_2 Joe broke the bat.

T-passive

       NP_2 + past + (be+en)   The bat was broken by

       + break + (by+NP_1)   Joe.

The superscripts 1 and 2 on the noun phrases are used to identify the noun phrases as they shift positions.

PASSIVE USES

The use of the passive form of a sentence often seems arbitrary. The sentences seem to have identical meanings either in their active or passive forms. It does seem, however, that it is possible to give the object more prominence by moving it to the front of the sentence, or, on the other hand, to subordinate the original subject by moving it to the end of the sentence or by deleting it. Remember that *by* plus the original subject noun phrase may be omitted. There are times, though, when the passive is necessary. These times are when the agent subject of the sentence is unknown or when an observer or writer wishes to remain anonymous:

3. The bank was robbed at 7:30 A.M.
4. The robbers were seen leaving in a van.

In example 3, the object noun phrase, *the bank,* warrants more prominence than the likely known agent subject which is *thieves,* or *robbers.* Example 4 shows the passive form often used in news-writing unless the reporter is given a *by-line.* It is for this reason that the passive is a quite commonly used form in newspapers and news magazines.

AUXILIARY STRUCTURES

In examples so far only *tense* has occurred in the auxiliary. However, the passive transformation will still work if other auxiliary elements are used.

1. NP_1 + present + will   April will buy a car.
   + buy + NP_2

T-passive

NP_2 + present + will   A car will be bought (by
+ (be+en) + buy +   April).
(by + NP_1)

2. NP_1 + past + (have+en)   Bill had seen the ele-
   + see + NP_2 phant.

T-passive

NP_2 + past + (have+en)   The elephant had been
+ (be+en) + see +   seen. (by Bill)
(by + NP_1)

3. NP_1 + past + (be+ing)   Jill was building a house.
   + build + NP_2

T-passive

NP_2 + past + (be+ing)   A house was being built.
+ (be+en) + build +   (by Jill)
(by + NP_1)

4. NP_1 + past + (Q) +   Bill had to feed the ele-
   feed + NP_2 phant.

T-passive

   NP_2 + past + (have to)   The elephant had to be
   + (be+en) + feed +   fed. (by Bill)
   (by + NP_1)

In examples 1 through 4 instances of the other auxiliary structures were used in sentences which were put through the passive
transformation. In all instances (be+en) will be inserted between the verb and any other existing auxiliary structures. The
parenthesis indicate that *by* plus agent subject is optional. Notice
in example 2 that the passive transformation produces two occurrences of the participle affix *en*.

Some people find that the combination of (be+ing) and one
of the other optional auxiliary elements is less than acceptable.
Consider the following examples which show the active and then
the passive forms of sentences which contain the auxiliary sequence tense + (modal) + (be+ing) and then tense + (have+en)
+ (be+ing):

5. The dog will be   The cat will be being
              (becomes)
   chasing the cat.   chased. (by the dog)

6. Someone has been   A house has been built.
   building a house.   (by someone)

AGREEMENT

If a passive transformation is applied to a sentence which has
a single subject and a plural object or the reverse, the auxiliary
structures must change to agree with the new subject.

1. Joe *builds* houses. (becomes) Houses *are* built. (by Joe)
2. They *were* building   A house *was* being built.
   a house.   (by them)
3. Jill *has* built   Houses have been built.
   houses.   (by Jill)

INDIRECT OBJECTS

Sentences which contain transitive verbs may have indirect as well as direct objects. Either of the two object noun phrases may shift as a part of T-passive.

1. NP_1 + past + give +   April gave *Jill* the *ball.*
   NP (ind. obj.) +
   NP (dir. obj.)

T-passive

NP (ind. obj.) + past +   Jill was given the ball.
(be+en) + give + NP   (by April)
(dir. obj.) + (by+NP_1)

[or]

NP (dir. obj.) + past +   The ball was given Jill.
(be+en) + give + NP   (by April)
(ind. obj.) + (by+NP_1)

TRANSITIVE VERB COMPLEMENTS

Not all sentences with transitive verb complements can be put through the passive transformation. The complement structure, whether infinitive phrase or participial phrase, must have a different subject noun phrase than that of the main sentence:

1. They found *Joe eating*   Joe was found eating an
   an apple.   apple. (by them)
   (becomes)
2. The teacher expected   Jill was expected to be-
   Jill to behave.   have. (by the teacher)
3. The children regarded   Joe was regarded as silly.
   Joe as silly.   (by the children)

Notice that the subject of the embedded sentence is shifted to the subject position and the infinitive or participial phrase remains in the complement position following the main verb.

YES/NO QUESTIONS

Passive sentences may be transformed into yes/no questions, but since a new auxiliary element has been added it may be helpful to reconsider the T-yes/no in terms of the passive sentence:

1. NP_1 + past + strike   Lightning struck the tree.
   + NP_2

T-passive

NP_2 + past + (be+en) +   The tree was struck by
strike + (by+NP_1)   lightning.

T-yes/no

past + be + NP_2 + en   Was the tree struck by
+ strike + (by+NP_1)   lightning?

Notice that the sequence *tense* + *be* was shifted to the beginning of the sentence as a result of T-yes/no. Also, the participle affix *en* was left in its original position.

GET. A common replacement for *be* in the passive transformation is *get*. It will substitute for *be,* producing the sequence (get+en). This form is frequently used but is considered to be quite informal. Consider these previously used examples with *get* substituted for *be*:

2. The tree *got* struck by lightning.
3. The house was *getting* built.
4. The bank *got* robbed.

PROBLEMS IN ACQUISITION

Passive sentences are relatively difficult structures for children to learn. Research with exceptional children (Power and Quigley, 1973) points out the very great difficulty that may be encountered with passive sentences. Hearing-impaired children have a tendency to process passive sentences in terms of the regular subject-verb-object sequence of active sentences. Apparently the markers of the passive (be+en) and *by* are not easily learned nor understood.

The most easily understood passive sentences are called *nonreversible.*

1. The house was cleaned by the man.

In this sentence the subject, verb, object interpretation is impossible since the house could not clean the man.

However, reversible passive forms are more difficult.

2. The boy was pushed by the girl.

Here, the first noun is much more easily interpreted as the agent subject. The most difficult passive sentences are those where the agent subject has been deleted. Apparently *by* is the most readily used clue to the interpretation of passive sentences.

EXERCISES

Perform the passive transformation on each of the following sentences:

1. The bird ate the worm. NP_1 + past + eat + NP_2

   T-passive

   NP_2 + past + (be+en) + eat + (by + NP_1)

   The worm was eaten. (by the bird)

2. The man was cutting down the tree. NP_1 + past + (be+ing) + cut down + NP_2

   T-passive

   NP_2 + past + (be+ing) + cut down + (by + NP_1)

   The tree was being cut down. (by the man)

3. The rain will help the plants. NP_1 + present + (will) + help + NP_2

   T-passive

   NP_2 + present + (will) + (be+en) + help + (by + NP_1)

   The plants will be helped. (by the rain)

Put this through the passive transformation in two ways. First, shift the direct object, then the indirect object.

4. The boy had given the girl the ball. NP_1 + past + (have+en) + give + the girl + NP_2

   T-passive
   (dir. obj.)

   The NP_2 + past + (have+ en) + (be+en) + give +

the girl + (by + NP$_1$)

The ball had been given the girl. (by the boy)

T-passive
(ind. obj.)

The girl + past + (have+ en) + (be+en) + give + the ball + (by + NP$_1$)

The girl had been given the ball. (by the boy)

5. The dog chased the cat.

NP$_1$ + past + chase + NP$_2$

T-passive

NP$_2$ + past + (be+en) + chase + (by + NP$_1$)

The cat was chased (by the dog)

6. The cat was catching fish.

NP$_1$ + past + (be+ing) + catch + NP$_2$

T-passive

NP$_2$ + past + (be+ing) + (be+en) + catch + (by + NP$_1$)

Fish were being caught. (by the cat)

POSSESSIVES

T HE POSSESSIVE, OR GENITIVE, takes the form of a noun phrase or pronoun form which indicates ownership or intimate relationship with the noun which follows. The possessive pronoun or noun, together with the noun which follows, constitute a more complex noun phrase.

The forms of the possessive pronouns were described in the chapter on pronouns. The possessive forms of regular nouns are quite simply formed by adding an *s* or *z* sound which is the same as the plural form of regular nouns. Regular, singularly possessive nouns are spelled with *'s*. The plural possessive form is spelled with *s'*.

HAVE

1. The boy has a dog.	(becomes)	The boy's dog
2. John has a bike.	(becomes)	John's bike
3. He has an idea.	(becomes)	His idea
4. The men have an airplane.	(becomes)	The men's airplane
5. April has two aunts.	(becomes)	April's two aunts

In the chapter on elementary sentence types the various shades of possession indicated with the verb *have* were discussed. These same shades of meaning are expressed in the derived possessive form.

TRANSITIVE VERBS

The possessive form is used to indicate relationships other than possession. In these cases a different simple sentence form will be the source for the possessive noun phrase:

1. Joe wrote poems.   Joe's poems
2. Jill painted pictures.   Jill's pictures
3. April builds houses.   April's houses

In these examples the meaning of the possessive reflects the work of a person. The work need not be in the possession of the person at all, though the same phrases would be used to indicate that relationship.

BE

Another possessive form is derived from the *be* sentence class which indicates purpose.

1. The store is for men.   The men's store
2. The school is for girls. The girl's school
3. The bike is for boys   The boy's bike

The possessive noun phrases derived from these base sentences are more like compound nouns than indicators of possession. They are descriptive of some referent. The possessive noun is used to indicate the kind of *store, school* or *bike,* etc. On the other hand, these same possessive noun phrases could have as their source *have* sentences and then the meaning would be quite different. Then *men's, girl's* and *boy's* would represent real owners rather than generic modifiers indicating purpose or type.

DEFINITE ARTICLE

The possessive noun phrase or pronoun functions as the determiner in the position held by the definite article. A transformation which is called the possessive transformation (T-poss) will embed the sentence containing the possessive relationships in the determiner position of the main sentence.

    1. Jack has a car.   (results in)

T-poss

    The car is old.   *Jack's* car is old.

    She has a farm.

T-poss

                             Her farm is small.

    The farm is small.

2. Mr. Smith has cows.

T-poss

Three of *Mr. Smith's*
cows give milk.

Three of *the* cows give milk.

OF

The preposition *of* is commonly used to indicate possession with essentially the same meaning as the previously-discussed possessive nouns. The following examples illustrate this parallel function:

1. The girl's dog   (or)   The dog of the girl
2. The man's house   (or)   The house of the man
3. The dog's tail   (or)   The tail of the dog

Notice that the possessive phrase follows rather than precedes the noun which indicates the thing possessed.

The *of* form may be preferred to the *'s* possessive when a series of possessives is used. Consider the following phrases in which both forms are used:

1. The desk of the first principal of the school
2. The school's first principal's desk

With nonanimate nouns the *of* phrase is more generally used in place of the *'s* form.

1. The middle of the room
2. The bottom of the hill
3. The front door of the houses

WITH

With was previously discussed with other prepositions. It has a number of uses among which is a function that is close to the possessives but not synonymous:

1. The boy *with a dog*
2. The door *with a red knob*
3. The cow *with a large hump*

As with nouns of the other possessive forms, these phrases are derived from *have* sentences. The following sentences are the logi-

cal source for the previous three examples:
  4. The boy has a dog.
  5. The door has a red knob.
  6. The cow has a large hump.

In examples 1 through 3 the *with* phrase seems to be secondary to the possible *of* phrases which could be produced from 4, 5 and 6 also. The *with* phrase seems to indicate possession in a more off-hand appositive fashion. It seems to add a clue to the identification of the modified noun.

NOUN REDUCTION

If sufficient context is available, the noun following the *'s* possessive can be deleted. Consider these examples where the noun is deleted:

  1. We bought cake at   We bought the cake
     Fred's bakery.   at Fred's.
  2. We borrowed *Mary's bike.*   We borrowed Mary's.

This reduction will add complexity in terms of the necessary use of context required to fill in the missing noun.

CHAPTER 18

THE THERE TRANSFORMATION

THE *there* under consideration in this chapter has been traditionally called an expletive. It is used at the beginning of some sentences which contain *be* either in the auxiliary or as the main verb. The word *there* is also used quite commonly as a one word adverb of place:

1. *There* is some food on the table.
2. *There* is a dog in the yard.
3. Joe found the dog *there*.

The first two sentences were produced by the *there* transformation (T-there). The third sentence contains *there* as an adverb of place.

The next two examples show the sentences from which examples 1 and 2 are derived by T-there:

4. *Some* food is on the   (becomes)   *There* is some food on table.   the table.
5. *A* dog is in the yard.   (becomes)   *There* is a dog in the yard.

Notice that the sentences which are to be transformed have some common features. Each has a nondefinite article in the subject noun phrase, each has a *be* verb, and each has an adverb of place.

Any of the nondefinite articles *a(n)*, *some* or the null form $(\emptyset)$ are generally requirements for this transformation. The negative particle *no* may be used in the article position of the subject noun phrase. *Any* may be used interchangeably with it after T-there has been performed:

6. No food is in the   (becomes)   There is *no* food in refrigerator.   the refrigerator.

117

[or]

There isn't *any* food in
the refrigerator.

The Ø article will permit the reduction of the *of* from pre-article constructions. We will, therefore, see structures such as the following which still meet the requirements for the transformation:

7. There are *many apples* on the tree.
8. There are *several boys* at school.

In all of the above examples, major stress in the sentence falls on the subject noun phrase which was placed after *be* by T-there. It is possible to produce sentences which have *there* at the initial position in the sentence and have a subject noun phrase containing a definite article which has shifted to the post *be* position. In this case, however, the word *there* will receive the major stress in the sentence.

9. There's *the* telephone. (ringing)
10. There are *those* bees in the attic.

The meaning is not the same as in the previous examples. These examples may illustrate a way of pointing out or calling attention to something.

The source of *be*, which is a required element to perform T-there, may be in the auxiliary structure (be+ing) :

11. Some boys *were*   (becomes)   There were some boys
    running in the hall.   running in the hall.
12. Some boys *were*   (becomes)   There were some boys
    flying a kite.   flying a kite.

The subject noun phrase again shifts to the position immediately following *be*. An adverb of place is not a requirement in these instances of T-there.

Another source of *be* is the passive transformation. Here the sequence (be+en) is added to the auxiliary, and if the nondefinite article condition is met, then a *there* transformation may apply:

13. A rock was thrown   (becomes)   There was a rock thrown
    at the bottle.   at the bottle.

14. Some trees were   (becomes)   There were some trees
    struck by lightning.   struck by lightning.

Be may be in an auxiliary structure as part of a quasi-modal. T-there may apply there as well.

15. Some girls were going (becomes) There were some girls
    to walk on the beach.   going to walk on the
                                     beach.

CONCLUSION

The alteration in normal word order and the fact that *there* is not an adverb of place can cause confusion. When T-there has applied to passive sentences, word order changes still further complicate an already complex structure.

EXERCISES

Apply T-there to the following sentences:

1. A boy is on the porch.   There is a boy on the
                                 porch.
2. Birds were flying   There were birds flying
   over the house.   over the house.
3. Some boys must have   There must have been
   been here.   some boys here.
4. A girl is riding   There is a girl riding
   her bike.   her bike.
5. Butterflies are caught   There are butterflies
   in the woods.   caught in the woods.
6. Many people are   There are many people
   visiting the park.   visiting the park.

RELATIVE CLAUSES

•••——•••

A RELATIVE CLAUSE IS PRODUCED by embedding one sentence in another sentence which has a noun in common with it. Relative clauses have frequently been called adjective clauses in that they modify or describe the common noun. The relative clause transformation (T-rel) is of considerable importance, not only because it is used to produce structures that are used with great frequency, but because it is the basis for some very important subsidiary transformations and structures. These subsidiary structures will be discussed in later chapters. The scope of relative clauses and the relative transformation itself are the subject of this chapter.

The italicized elements in the following examples illustrate the relative clauses which have been embedded by T-rel:

1. The boy *who has red hair* hit Pete.
2. The boy likes dogs *that are big*.

Notice that each relative clause started with a relative pronoun. In these examples they were *who* and *that*. The most common relative pronouns are *who, which* and *that* along with the inflected forms of *who (whom* and *whose)*.

The sentences which were transformationally joined to produce examples 1 and 2 are illustrated in the following examples:

3. The *boy hit* Pete.

T-rel

the boy *who has red hair* hit Pete.

The *boy* has red hair.
4. The boy likes *dogs*.

120

T-rel

The boy likes dogs
that are big.

Some *dogs* are big.

The nouns which are common to both the main sentences and the sentences which are to be embedded by T-rel are italicized.

Notice that by T-rel the relative pronoun replaces the entire noun phrase in the embedded sentence, and the relative clause is positioned following the common noun in the main sentence.

SHARED NOUNS

Nouns are shared between the main and embedded sentences. The function of these nouns in their respective sentences can be in any of the possible noun phrase locations that sentences have. The common noun may have the same function in both sentences or they may have different functions. The following examples illustrate the relative transformation as it is performed on sentences with varying noun functions. The first to be considered will have parallel functions of the noun phrases. In other words, the noun in the main and the embedded sentence have the same function:

1. The *boy* ran home.

T-rel

The boy *who caught a fish* ran home.

The *boy* caught a fish.

2. Father cooked the *fish*.

T-rel

Father cooked the fish *which the boy caught.*

The boy caught a *fish*.

In example 1 the shared nouns in both the main and embedded sentences function in subject noun phrases. The shared nouns in example 2 function in direct object noun phrases. Notice that in example 1 the relative clause is embedded in the middle of the sentence while in example 2 it is at the end of the main sentence.

The relative pronoun *which* will be used with nonhuman and nonanimate nouns.

In the next examples the shared nouns will have differing functions in their main and embedded sentences:

3. The *boy* ran home.

T-rel

The boy *that the girl hit* ran home.

The girl hit the *boy*.

4. The dog bit the *boy*.

T-rel

The dog bit the boy *who ran home.*

The *boy* ran home.

In example 3 the shared noun is in the subject of the main sentence and the object of the embedded sentence. The shared nouns in example 4 function in the object of the main sentence and the subject of the embedded sentence. Notice from the examples so far the shared noun in the main sentence controls the position of the relative clause. Also, the shared noun in the embedded sentence is replaced by an appropriate relative pronoun. The relative pronoun will be shifted to the front of the relative clause if the noun it replaces is in a position other than the subject.

So far the positions of the shared nouns which have been considered were in subjects and direct objects only. The next examples contain instances of shared nouns in indirect objects and prepositional phrases:

5. The boy gave the *dog* a bone.

T-rel

The boy gave the dog *which was happy* a bone.

The *dog* was happy.

6. The girl lived by the *lady*.

T-rel

The girl lived by the
lady *that had a truck.*

The *lady* had a truck.
7. The boy saw the *rabbit.*
T-rel

The boy saw the rabbit
that there was a tree by.

There was a tree by
the *rabbit.*

[or]
The boy saw the rabbit
by which there was a
tree.

In example 5 the shared noun appears in an indirect object in the main sentence and the subject of the embedded sentence. In example 6 the noun appears in the object of a preposition in the main sentence and the subject of the embedded sentence. In example 7 the noun is in the object of the main sentence and the object of the preposition of the embedded sentence.

Notice that in example 7 there are two relative clause forms. When the shared noun is in the object of a preposition, the relative pronouns *whom* or *which* can replace the noun phrase object of the preposition and the sequence *preposition* plus *relative pronoun* will be shifted to the front of the relative clause form. The relative pronoun *that* cannot shift with a preposition.

Among their other uses, *when* and *where* may be used as relative pronouns. *When* is used when the shared noun of the embedded sentence is in an adverb of time, and *where* is used when the shared noun is in an adverb of place:

8. He lives in the *town.*
T-rel

He lives in the town
where he was born.

He was born in the *town.* [or]
He lives in the town
in which he was born.

9. He remembers the *day*.

T-rel

He remembers the day
when you were born.

You were born on that *day*.

[or]

He remembers the day
on which you were born.

Notice that *where* or *when* replaces the entire prepositional phrase containing the shared noun in the embedded sentences. Since the shared nouns of the embedded sentences were in prepositional phrases, the alternate form of the relative clause may be used. In this form *which* replaces the noun phrase and moves with the preposition to the front of the clause. The less formal form leaves the preposition at the end of the clause.

The relative pronoun *whose* is used to replace possessive nouns or pronouns:

10. The *boy* bought a bike.

T-rel

The boy *whose father
gave him fifty dollars*
bought a bike.

The *boy's father* gave
him fifty dollars.

11. They helped the boy.

T-rel

They helped the boy
whose father they found.

They found the *boy's*
father.

Notice that the relative pronoun *whose* replaces the determiner and the possessive noun or pronoun. As in example 11, the sequence *whose* plus the possessed noun will be shifted to the front of the relative clause when it is in a position other than the subject.

RESTRICTIVE AND NONRESTRICTIVE

The relative clauses presented to this point are called restrictive relative clauses. They are used to identify or restrict the meaning of the noun which they follow. The nonrestrictive type is not used to identify or restrict meaning. It is used simply to add information and can be omitted without changing the information or meaning provided by the main sentence. Consider the following sentences, the first with a restrictive relative clause and the second with a nonrestrictive form:

1. The girl *that has red hair* hit the boy.
2. April, *who looks like Jill,* has a chicken.

Nonrestrictive relative clauses are set off by commas. In speech the nonrestrictive clause is marked by a different intonation pattern than the restrictive form. Also, the boundaries of the clause are marked by more distinct pauses.

The relative pronoun *that* cannot be used in restrictive clauses. If it is used, then the clause is restrictive. Proper nouns are normally followed by nonrestrictive relatives since they don't ordinarily require further identification. It is sometimes necessary to further specify or identify even proper nouns, so in these instances the proper noun will be preceded by a definite article and the clause will be restrictive:

3. The Jerry Ford *that I know* is a fireman.
4. The April *that looks like Jill* has a chicken.

Notice that since the relative clauses are restrictive, the relative pronoun *that* may be used.

When the relative pronoun replaces a noun used in the object, indirect object or object of preposition of the relative clauses, the relative pronoun may be deleted in restrictive clauses:

5. The girl *Joe met* had a bike.
6. The bike *Joe bought* is a ten-speed.

SPLIT ANTECEDENTS

Usually a relative clause immediately follows the shared noun in the main sentence. However, a relative clause can be moved to the end of the main sentence. Consider these examples showing the normal position and then the sentence end position:

1. A boy *who had a*   (becomes)   A boy came to school
 rabbit came to school.   *who had a rabbit.*
2. The girl *who has*   The girl lives next
 a snake lives next   door *who has a*
 door.   *snake.*

SENTENCE ANTECEDENTS

The relative clauses which have been presented to this point have shared nouns or nominal forms with the main sentence. In some forms, however, the relative clause seems to refer to an entire sentence rather than to the single noun in a sentence:

1. Joe broke a window, *which his mother didn't like.*
2. The truck splashed through a puddle, *which got Joe all wet.*
3. The girl goes to the dentist every year, *which is a good idea.*

This form of relative clause is nonrestrictive. A comma is used to indicate the pause which separates this relative clause from the main sentence.

ACQUISITION OF RELATIVE CLAUSES

Amy Sheldon (1972) studied the acquisition of relative clauses by children between the ages of three and three-fourths and five and one-half. She studied four kinds of clauses based on the functions of the nouns shared between the main and relative clauses. The shared nouns in the sentences she studied had the following forms: subject-subject, subject-object, object-subject and object-object. Her findings indicate that if the nouns have a parallel function in their respective clauses, they were learned more readily by children in this age group.

Quigley, Smith and Wilbur (1974) studied the comprehension of relative clauses which were embedded in the middle and at the end of sentences. The populations which they studied were deaf children from ten to eighteen and normal children from eight to ten. Their findings suggest that both deaf and hearing subjects have more difficulty understanding relative clauses when the relative pronoun replaces the object of the embedded sentence than when it replaces the subject. Also, both groups have much greater difficulty when relative clauses are in the middle of a sentence than when they are in the final position.

They also point out that deaf children tend to misinterpret sentences which contain relative clauses. They apparently do this by trying to fit these more complex sentences into a simple subject-verb-object-word order.

EXERCISES

Perform the relative transformation on the following sentence pairs. Embed the second sentence as the relative clause.

1. The girl has a dog.

T-rel

The girl saw the wreck.	The girl who saw the wreck has a dog.

2. Mother baked the cake

T-rel

The cake is on the table.	Mother baked the cake that is on the table.

3. The doctor gave medicine to the boy.

T-rel

The boy was sick.	The doctor gave medicine to the boy who was sick.

4. They went to the city.

T-rel

The play is in the city.	They went to the city where the play is. [or] They went to the city in which the play is.

5. The girl bought the car.

T-rel

The boy visited the girl's sister.	The girl whose sister the boy visited bought the car.

6. The boy drives a tractor.

T-rel

The boy's father has a horse.	The boy whose father has a horse drives a tractor.

7. Autumn is a season.

T-rel

Trees lose their leaves in autumn.	Autumn is a season when trees lose their leaves. [or] Autumn is a season in which trees lose their leaves.

8. Father bought the house.

T-rel

The Smiths had lived in the house.	Father bought the house where the Smiths had lived. [or] Father bought the house in which the Smiths had lived.

9. The ball was given to the boy.

T-rel

The girl was kissed by the boy.	The ball was given to the boy by whom the girl was kissed. [or] The ball was given to the boy who the girl was kissed by.

10. Mother gave candy to the baby.

T-rel

The girl bought the baby a rattle.	Mother gave candy to the baby who(m) the girl bought a rattle.

NOUN MODIFIERS

T HE VARIOUS MODIFIERS of nouns are derived from underlying sentences that also contained those nouns and which make some assertions about them. All of the noun modifiers will have as a first step in their history a sentence that was embedded by a relative clause transformation.

PHRASES USED AS NOUN MODIFIERS

Consider the following pair of sentences:

1. The boy *who was wearing a red cap* pulled the cat's tail.
2. The boy *wearing a red cap* pulled the cat's tail.

The italicized portion of sentence 1 is a relative clause. The italicized *ing* phrase in sentence 2 is sometimes called an adjectival phrase. Sentence 2 is derived from sentence 1 by the deletion of the sequence relative pronoun, tense and *be*. This deletion transformation is possible any time that the sequence relative pronoun tense and *be* occurs. The *be* may come from the auxiliary (be+ing), the passive transformation, or *be* as the main verb.

ING PHRASES

The *ing* or participial phrases are derived from relative clauses. The deletion of relative pronoun, tense and *be* then changes the relative clause to the phrase form:

1. The girl *running down the street* is Mary.
2. The man *waiting in the hall* has a package.
3. April, *feeling much better,* went to school.

In sentence 3 the *ing* phrase came from a nonrestrictive relative clause. Notice that the intonation pattern remains the same and the commas are retained to indicate pauses.

The following pair of sentences illustrates how the negative appears as the relative clause is reduced to the phrase form:

4. The boy *who isn't riding a bike* is Fred.
5. The boy *not riding a bike* is Fred.

Some *ing* phrases are more likely to be produced by a variation of the relative clause deletion transformation. This is because some of the sentences embedded by T-rel have different auxiliary structures or are unlikely to have had (be+ing) in their auxiliaries, The following sentences contain *ing* phrases which were produced by deleting the relative pronoun and replacing tense with *ing*.

6. The boy, *having slept late,* missed the bus.
7. The dog, *being quite old,* ran slowly.
8. The girl, *knowing all the answers,* felt pleased.

PASSIVE PARTICIPLE PHRASES

When passive sentences are embedded as relative clauses, they produce the sequence relative pronoun, tense and *be*. This sequence is deletable, and when it is, it produces participle phrases such as the following:

1. The horse, *purchased by the girl,* is gentle.
2. The tree, *blown down by the wind,* was a cedar.
3. The fish, *caught by the children,* were bass.

PREPOSITIONAL PHRASES

Prepositional phrases which are adverbials of place may be used as noun modifiers. Prepositional phrases which are adverbs of place may appear in relative clauses with *be* verbs such as the following:

1. The house *that is on the hill* is mine.
2. The girl *who is in the boat* is fishing.

APPOSITIVES

Noun phrases following *be* in relative clauses may appear as modifiers called appositives if the relative deletion transformation is performed. Sentence 1 shows the relative clause form and sentence 2 shows the appositive form:

1. The man, *who was a detective,* caught the thief.
2. The man, *a detective,* caught the thief.

Other examples of appositives are

3. Helen, *a friend of Mary,* came to visit.
4. The car, *a Ford,* had a flat tire.

ADJECTIVES WITH PREPOSITIONAL PHRASES

Adjectives with prepositional phrases may follow *be* in relative clauses such as

1. The boy *who was happy about his grades* skipped home.
2. The man *who was exhausted from the trip* fell into bed.

By performing the relative deletion transformation on sentences 1 and 2, the following sentences are produced:

3. The boy, *happy about his grades,* skipped home.
4. The man, *exhausted from the trip,* fell into bed.

THE NOUN MODIFIER TRANSFORMATION

The noun modifiers examined so far have been in phrase forms. After the relative deletion transformation these phrases remained in the position following the nouns that they modify. However, when the deletion transformation leaves a single word in the modifier position following the noun, the word frequently must be shifted to the position between the determiner and the noun. This transformation is called the noun modifier transformation (T-noun modifier), and it follows the relative clause deletion transformation. The following sentences show the three stages in this sequence:

1. The boy who was happy skipped down the hall. (by T-rel)

T-relative deletion

*The boy *happy* skipped down the hall.

T-noun modifier

The *happy* boy skipped down the hall.

Notice that the deletion transformation does not leave a grammatical form in step 2 of the example. The noun modifier transformation is obligatory and places the adjective in the noun modifier position before the noun in the last step.

The first example shows how an adjective was shifted by the noun modifier transformation. Parts of speech other than adjectives may be shifted by the noun modifier transformation following the same sequence of operations. The next two sets of examples show how a verb may be shifted by T-noun modifier.

    2. She met some children *who were laughing.* (by T-rel)
T-relative deletion
        She met some children *laughing.*
T-noun modifier
        She met some *laughing* children.

    3. The snow which was melting covered the garden. (by T-rel)
T-relative deletion
        The snow *melting,* covered the garden.
T-noun modifier
        The *melting* snow covered the garden.

Passive verbs may also undergo the noun modifier transformation.

    4. The game which was interrupted was tied. (by T-rel)
T-relative deletion
        *The game *interrupted* was tied.
T-noun modifier
        The *interrupted* game was tied.

Verbs followed by adverbials of manner can be optionally shifted together by T-noun modifier.

    5. The path *which was followed carefully* went uphill.
T-relative deletion
        The path *followed carefully* went uphill.
T-noun modifier
        The *carefully followed* path went uphill.

One-word adverbs of place may optionally be shifted by T-noun modifiers. The transformation will change phrases like *the closet downstairs, a school nearby* and *the light outside* to *the downstairs closet, a nearby school, the outside light.*

Nouns may be shifted to the noun modifier slot between the determiner and the noun. The scope of nouns as noun modifiers is somewhat more complex than for the other noun modifiers. These noun modifiers may originate in more than one sentence type while the resultant forms give no obvious syntactic clue as to what the originating sentence might have been. The sentence sources are quite often from forms of simple *be* verb sentences. The following phrases show nouns in the noun modifier slot which come from slightly different *be* verb sentence sources: *A kitchen table, a history book, a paint can, an April day.*

The following sentences are the likely sources of these nouns used as noun modifiers:

6. A table is for a kitchen.
7. A book is about history.
8. A can is for paint.
9. A day is in April.

The preposition continued in each of the above sentences is apparently erased when the noun shifts by T-noun modifier.

MULTIPLE NOUN MODIFIERS

There is no limit to the number of noun modifiers which can be derived from the sequence of transformations T-rel, T-deletion, T-noun modifier. The primary limitations are stylistic acceptability and the short-term memory limitation of the average speaker-listener:

1. John bought the *banged up, old rusty, yellow pickup* truck.

Ing verbs and passive verbs can be added indefinitely:

2. The toy was a sleeping, walking, talking doll.
3. The tired, dejected, dispirited, beaten team went to the locker room.

Multiple nouns may appear as modifiers in noun phrases, too. However, the order in which they appear is critical. Each noun in a sequence of nouns modifies the next one, so, in the phrase the *apple crate nail salesman,* the order is rigidly fixed or the phrase would have an entirely different meaning or become nonsense.

Table VI

ORDER OF ADJECTIVES

Characteristics	Size	Shape	Temperature & Humidity	Age	Color	Origin	Head Noun
	short	stocky				Arabian	horse
beautiful	small				white	Persian	cat
			hot, humid			Tropical	climate
witty			warm		color-ful		personality

Adjectives, too, will make multiple appearances, but their order is even more restricted. The position in the modifying order of the adjectives is quite rigid in the phrase *an unusual long old yellow truck*. Brown (1965) suggests the sequence shown in Table VI for the order of adjectives in noun phrases.

Various adjective modifier sequences are illustrated in the frame to help define each adjective slot.

In any event, if a noun occurs in a sequence of noun modifiers, it must appear in the position just before the modified noun. In phrases such as *the red kitchen chair, the new history book, the stalled pickup truck* or *the idling motorcycle motor* you will notice that the noun cannot change position with any of the other various modifying words.

CONCLUSION

Noun modifiers have all of the complexity and semantic value of the structures from which they were derived. For example, passive verbs used as modifiers came from passive sentences which have demonstrated difficulty. The transformations which produced the various modifiers greatly reduce or obscure many syntactic clues as to the nature of the sentences of their origin. The modifiers may be short, but this shortness belies the complexity of their origin's structure and derivation.

CHAPTER 21

NOUN CLAUSES

N OUN CLAUSES ARE SENTENCES which are used in place of noun phrases. The transformation which embeds sentences as noun phrases is relatively simple. The noun clause sentence is embedded in an empty noun phrase position in the main sentence. This transformation is called the noun clause transformation (T-noun clause) :

1. He knew *that Jill won the prize.*
2. The boy guessed *what the right answer was.*
3. The girl realized *that it was lunch time.*

Noun clauses are often introduced by *that.* Others are introduced by the various question words *when, where, who, what, how, why,* etc. The words *if* and *whether* are used in certain cases as introductory words also.

IN THE VERB PHRASE

Noun clauses commonly appear in the verb phrase as direct objects:

1. John heard *(that) Fred is a scout.*
2. April forgot *(that) it was Saturday.*

The introductory *that* is optional when noun clauses are used as direct objects. The verbs which accept noun clauses as direct objects include *think, know, believe, find, learn, hear, ask, say, demand,* etc. The number of verbs which take noun clause objects is fairly extensive. A good many suggest some mental or communicative activity.

Noun clauses can function as noun phrases following *be* when the subject nouns are words like *fact, idea, thought, notion, belief,* etc.:

135

3. The truth was *(that) Joe didn't have any money.*
4. The belief is *(that) cats have nine lives.*
That is optional when noun clauses follow *be* as well.

AS SUBJECTS

Use of noun clauses as subjects is more common to formal writing than to general use. More frequently the subject noun clause will be replaced by *it* and the clause repositioned in the verb phrase:

1. *That he was late* surprised the teacher.
2. *It* surpised the teacher *that he was late.*
3. *Why he left early* was a mystery.
4. *It* was a mystery *why he left early.*

Noun clauses appear as the subject of copulative verbs, *have,* and transitive verbs which take abstract nouns as subjects.

Noun clauses may be positioned in the subject position of passive sentences. When this situation occurs the clause may be replaced by *it* and repositioned at the end of the sentence.

5. *That the ceremony caused the rain* was believed (by the natives).
6. *It* was believed (by the natives) *that the ceremony caused the rain.*

AS OBJECTS OF PREPOSITIONS

Noun clauses can function as objects of prepositions. The question word clauses seem to be the most commonly used after prepositions:

1. They can see *from where their house is.*
2. He left *after what the policeman told him.*
3. He put the food *in what looked like an antique cupboard.*

QUESTION WORD CLAUSES

Sentences embedded as noun clauses of the question word form have one element replaced by the appropriate question word (who, what, when, how, why, how often, etc.). The question word is shifted to the front of the clause as in the regular *wh* question transformation:

1. I know *why he came.*
2. He discovered *where the treasure was.*
3. He learned *how he could fix his bike.*

Question words will combine with *ever* to form introductory words such as *whatever, whoever, wherever,* etc.:

4. *Whoever you invite* is fine.
5. He likes *whatever Fred likes.*
6. *Whoever rubs the lamp* shall have *whatever they wish.*

Yes/no questions may be embedded as noun clauses. *If* is the introductory word for most yes/no questions, but *whether* is used if the embedded yes/no question contains the conjunction *or:*

7. Joe wondered *if he would get a bike for Christmas.*
8. Fred asked *if Joe would come to his party.*
9. The girl asked *whether she could go or not.*

The number of verbs which accept yes/no noun clauses is fairly restricted. The verb *ask* quite frequently occurs in this way in a form called indirect discourse. Indirect discourse forms will be discussed in more detail in a later chapter. The verbs *wonder, decide* and *know* also permit yes/no noun clauses as a direct object.

NOUN CLAUSES AFTER ADJECTIVES

Noun clauses which are introduced by *that* may occur with adjectives followed by copulative verb forms:

1. He was *happy that his mother came.*
2. They were *anxious that they arrived on time.*
3. They seemed *startled that the cow jumped over the moon.*

The clause forms shown above form causal relationships with the main sentences. *Because* could be substituted for *that* in each of these sentences without changing the meaning. The restrictions on this formulation are rather strict. The copulative verb requires a human or animate subject, and the adjective must be descriptive of an emotional state.

Another small group of adjectives including *sure, confident, certain, conscious, skeptical, aware,* etc., may be followed by noun clauses in noncausal relationships:

4. He was *aware that Pete was his friend.*

5. They were *certain that she would win.*

Here again the main sentences require a human or animate subject, a copulative verb and certain adjectives denoting a mental state or activity. *Because* will not substitute for *that* in these sentences.

NOUN CLAUSES WITH NOUNS

Noun clauses may be used as noun modifiers. Their derivation is likely the same as other noun modifier forms. The result, however, is an exceedingly complex structure.

1. *The notion that they would ride an elephant* seemed strange.
2. *The belief that the dish ran away with the spoon* persisted.
3. They had *an argument that congressional salaries should be reduced.*

The nouns which these clauses modify denote mental activity. Others include *fact, idea, decision, concept, excuse,* etc.

Clauses of this type can be shifted from the modifying position to the end of the main sentence. The clauses in sentences 1 and 2 are shifted in this manner in the following examples:

4. The notion seemed strange *that they would ride an elephant.*
5. The belief persisted *that the dish ran away with the spoon.*

THE SUBJUNCTIVE WITH NOUN CLAUSES

The subjunctive verb form *were* appears in some noun clauses when the meaning is intended to be doubtful or hypothetical.

1. I wish that I *were* a giant.

The other subjunctive form occurs in noun clauses when the meaning is related to a requested action. In these examples the verb of the noun clause will carry no indication of tense or agreement.

2. He asked that you *be* quiet.
3. They ordered that the mess *be* cleaned up.
4. Joe demanded that Pete *apologize.*

CONCLUSION

Noun phrases comprised of single nouns with their determiner structures are relatively simple to process as subjects or objects of sentences. However, when the noun phrase function is taken by an entire sentence, itself containing the variety of possible sentence relationships, the difficulty of the new sentence is considerably increased. The further shifting of the clauses and the *it* replacement will further complicate these structures.

CHAPTER 22

NOMINALIZING TRANSFORMATIONS

Sentences may be transformed into abstract nouns. These transformations may alter the appearance of the sentence substantially, but the resultant nouns will be essentially synonymous with their sentence antecedents.

FOR ... TO

The first transformation (T-for . . . to) under consideration nominalizes a sentence by placing the preposition *for* in front of the subject and replacing *tense* with *to:*

1. The boy ran. (becomes by T-for . . . to) *For* the boy to run

The only auxiliary structures which will not survive T-for . . . to are the traditional modals. However, any of the quasi-modals will survive the transformation:

2. The boy is running. (becomes) For the boy to be running
3. The girl has run. (becomes) For the girl to have run
4. The boy is going to run. (becomes) For the boy to be going to run

When the subject of the sentence is a personal pronoun, it will change to the objective form as a result of T-for/to:

5. He left. (becomes) For him to leave

Nouns produced by T-for . . . to have a rather restricted range of uses. One use is as the subject of sentences with *be* verbs or verbs which take abstract noun as subjects:

6. *For John to be late* was strange.
7. *For Pete to pay the bills* is important.
8. *For the boys to be late* angers the teacher.

140

9. *For anyone to break* the balloon was mean.

10. *For someone to help Fred* was kind.

In examples 11 and 12 the subject of the nominalized sentence is not particularly necessary. In such instances the preposition *for* together with the subject may be deleted:

11. *To break the balloon* was mean.

12. *To help Fred* was kind.

Whenever the subject is not important or when surrounding context is sufficient to identify the subject, *for* plus the subject are deletable.

When nominalized sentences of this type occur as subjects they may be replaced by *it*, then shifted to the end of the sentence:

13. *It* was strange *for John to be late.*

14. *It* angers the teacher *for the boys to be late.*

15. *It* was mean *to break the balloon.*

Sentences transformed by for/to can occur as complements after *be:*

16. The coat is *for you to wear.*

17. The vacation's purpose was *for us to have a good time.*

Here again the sequence *for* plus the subject may be deleted if there is sufficient context. The deletion ordinarily must take place if the subject in the embedded sentence is repetitious of a noun in the main sentence:

18. Joe's idea was *(for Joe) to have fun.*

When sentences transformed by for/to are used as complements after *be,* they usually imply purpose or reason. It is quite likely that they overlap the simple sentence frame where *be* can be followed by an adverb of purpose which was discussed in the second chapter:

19. The coat is *for you.*

20. You wear the coat.   (becomes by T-for. . . .to) For you to wear the coat.

And by embedding 20 in 19 through the use of T-for/to we have

21. The coat is *for you to wear (the coat).*

Notice that the redundant noun phrase *the coat* must be deleted from the embedded structure.

The for/to nominalization may be used to indicate purpose,

reason or cause quite generally. As in the other examples, the redundant subject with *for* will be deleted:

22. Joe left early *(for Joe) to start on his vacation.*
23. *(For the bird) to get the worm,* the bird got up early.

Notice that the phrases used in this way may be placed at either end of the main sentence. Also, the words *in order* may precede the *for . . . to* constructions:

24. *In order for him to win,* Fred must lose twice.
25. Joe left early *in order to start his vacation.*

In the last chapter, noun clauses which began with question words such as *how, what, who, why,* etc., were discussed. This noun clause transformation together with T-for . . . to is responsible for the very complex noun phrases such as *how to patent your inventions, what to wear to camp, when to visit the national parks,* etc. These structures occur quite commonly as titles as well as in general discourse.

POSSESSIVE . . . ING

Nouns produced by the possessive . . . ing transformation (T-poss . . . ing) are used more flexibly than those produced by T-for . . . to. They may occur in any NP position where an abstract noun is grammatical. The essential features of the transformation are the change to the possessive form of the subject and the replacement of tense with *ing*. Again, as with T-for . . . to, the only auxiliary elements which will not survive this transformation are the traditional modals:

1. The boy ran (becomes by T-poss . . . ing)

   The boy's running
2. Pete has run   (becomes)   Pete's having run
3. He has to go   (becomes)   His having to go

Notice that in example 3 the personal pronoun changes to the possessive pronoun form as a result of T-poss . . . ing.

The next examples show the *poss . . . ing* structures in various noun phrase positions:

4. *Joe's driving* surprised the policeman.
5. The mechanic understood *the motor's rattling.*
6. He was alerted by *the dog's barking.*

Just as with the *for . . . to* structures, the subject is deletable if it is unneeded or redundant. In this instance the possessive noun or pronoun is deleted.

7. *(Someone's) setting a new record* was a surprise.

8. He opened the can by *(his) using a knife.*

If the sentence being transformed by *poss . . . ing* is transitive, an optional variation is possible. The preposition *of* may be inserted before the direct object:

9. Joe hit the ball.   (becomes by T-poss . . . ing)

> Joe's hitting the ball
> [or]
> Joe's hitting *of* the ball

10. They bought the car. (becomes) Their buying the car
> [or]
> Their buying of the car

The possessive can be formed by use of the preposition *of,* so many of the poss-ing transformations discussed to this point could have this possessive form:

11. The boy ran.   (becomes) The boy's running
> [or]
> The running of the boy

12. The lion growled.   The lion's growling
> [or]
> The growling of the lion

OTHER NOMINALIZED FORMS

The following examples show the transformation of sentences by T-poss . . . ing, then the other nominalized forms that the same sentence can have.

1. Joe is tall.   (becomes) Joe's being tall
> [or]
> Joe's tallness

[or]

The tallness of Joe

2. Joe arrived.   (becomes)   Joe's arriving

[or]

Joe's arrival

[or]

The arrival of Joe

In example 1 the verb *be* may be deleted entirely and the noun form of the adjective, if it has one, is formed. In example 2 the verb may change to a noun form through one of the various suffixes rather than to the *ing* form.

CONCLUSION

Nominalized sentences form abstract singular nouns. The derivation of these forms alters the syntactic form and the sentence origins of these structures. Additionally, various components may be reduced under certain conditions. The double problem of abstractness and syntactic complexity makes these structures quite difficult. It is likely these reasons account for the absence of such structures from the language of many handicapped children.

EXERCISES

Transform the following sentences by T-for . . . to:

1. John has a dog.   (for John) to have a dog
2. The girl is sad.   (for the girl) to be sad
3. He had gone to the store.   (for him) to have gone to the store
4. The birds are flying.   (for the birds) to be flying
5. The boy had to eat mashed carrots.   (for the boy) to have to eat mashed carrots

In the next exercises, transform sentence (a) by T-for . . . to then embed it in the NP of sentence (b) :

1. (a) The dog howled.   (for the dog) to howl
   (b) NP is unusual   (for the dog) to howl is unusual

2. (a) We go to the park.   (for us) to go to the park
   (b) NP is fun   (for us) to go to the park is
                                    fun

Transform the following sentences by T-poss . . . ing:

1. The baby cried.   (the baby's) crying
2. The lady watches his   (the lady's) watching his
   swimming.   swimming
                                         [or]
                                    (the lady's) watching of his
                                    swimming
3. Father cooked supper.   (father's) cooking supper
                                         [or]
                                    father's cooking *of* supper
4. The woman had been sad.   (the woman's having been
                                    sad)

Transform sentence (a) by T-poss . . . ing and then embed it
in the NP of sentence (b) :

1. (a) Joe drives.   (Joe's) driving
   (b) NP wastes a lot of gas.   (Joe's) driving wastes a lot
                                    of gas
2. (a) Joe snores.   (Joe's) snoring
   (b) Fred was awakened by   Fred   was   awakened   by
        NP.   (Joe's) snoring

Identify the sentences from which the following nominalized
forms were derived. (Either present or past tense is correct.)

1. The boy's climbing of the tree. The boy climbed the tree.
2. The building's swaying.   The building swayed.
3. John's refusal of the job.   John refused the job.
4. The tree's width.   The tree was wide.
5. The snake's being long.   The snake was long.

CLEFT SENTENCES

THERE ARE TWO TRANSFORMATIONS which alter the word order of sentences in order to emphasize certain parts. One of these transformations divides the sentence over a frame containing *be*. The other transformation applies to already complex sentences and involves *it* replacement and movement of subject clauses and phrases.

WH...BE...

Given a sentence like *The cat caught a mouse,* we can divide it in three ways to emphasize the subject, the object or the entire verb phrase. All three of the divisions will be made over the sentence frame *what ... be ....* The following examples illustrate this cleft transformation (T-cleft) and the emphasis of the three sentence parts:

1. What caught a mouse *was the cat.* (subject)
2. What the cat caught was *a mouse.* (object)
3. What the cat did was *catch a mouse.* (verb phrase)

The subject of the cleft sentences becomes a question word noun clause. The interrogative word in fact represents or replaces the emphasized part which follows *be* in the main sentence frame. In example 3, where the verb phrase was emphasized, notice that the question word noun clause has the form of a *what-do* question. In this case *what* and *do* represent the emphasized verb phrase which is placed after *be* in the main sentence.

The *wh* word which begins the cleft sentence may be any of the varieties of question words which are appropriate replacements for any of the sentence parts to be emphasized. Consider

146

the various divisions by points of emphasis on this sentence—*Jill took Pete to school on Monday.*

4. Who took Pete to school on Monday was *Jill.* (subject)
5. Whom Jill took to school on Monday was *Pete.* (object)
6. Where Jill took Pete on Monday was *to school.* (adverb of place)
7. When Jill took Pete to school was *on Monday.* (adverb of time)
8. What Jill did was *take Pete to school on Monday.* (verb phrase)

The following example illustrates the use of *why* and *how* as question word replacements for the cleft transformation. T-cleft is applied to the sentence—*Joe went to work by bus to save gas.*

9. How Joe went to work to save gas was *by bus.* (means)
10. Why Joe went to work by bus was *to save gas.* (reason)

Adjectives may also be emphasized. If we apply T-cleft to the sentence *Joe is tall,* we get

11. What Joe is is *tall.*

Another fairly common idiomatic replacement for *what* in some cleft sentences is the word pair *all that.* The following example substitutes *all that* for *what* in the cleft transformation of the sentence—*The boys could see two eyes.*

12. *All that* the boys could see was two eyes.

CLEFT MOVEMENT

It was mentioned in previous chapters that certain structures in subject positions before *be* could be replaced by *it* and then moved to the end of the sentence. This same *it* replacement and movement is possible with the cleft sentences which were just discussed. The following sentences show the cleft sentences before and after *it* replacement and movement:

1. What caught a mouse   It was *the cat* that caught
(becomes)
was the cat.   a mouse.

2. What the cat caught   It was *a mouse* that the cat
(becomes)
was *a mouse.*   caught.

3. Where Jill took Pete was *to school*.	It was *to school* that Jill took Pete.
4. Why he took the bus was *to save gas*.	It was *to save gas* that he took the bus.
5. Who took Pete to school was *Jill*.	It was *Jill* who took Pete to school.

Notice that the question word which introduces the cleft sentence may change to *that* after the clause is moved. Notice, also, that the same point of emphasis is retained after this transformation.

The other forms of this transformation were briefly introduced in the chapters on noun clauses and the chapter on nominalizing transformations. The following sentences have noun clauses as subjects which are replaced by *it* and then moved to the end of the main sentence:

6. That Fred was late was unusual.	It was unusual that Fred was late.
7. What he wanted to wear was his business.	It was his business what he wanted to wear.
8. How he earned his money was dangerous.	It was dangerous how he earned his money.

Notice that when this transformation applies to sentences with noun clause subjects, but which are not the result of T-cleft, the question words are retained after *it* replacement and movement. This transformation in either case is sometimes called the *extraposition* transformation.

CONCLUSION

The cleft transformation serves to emphasize specific sentence elements. The original meaning of the sentence remains through the cleft transformation, but the syntactic complexity is greatly increased. The complexity is still further compounded by the transposition of the subject clause and its replacement by *it*. This complexity makes such structures among the most difficult to acquire and among the last learned. For anyone interested in further study of cleft sentences, they are referred to the article by Akmajian (1970) on this topic.

EXERCISES

Apply the cleft transformation to the following sentences. Emphasize the underlined elements.

1. Joe *left*.	What Joe did was leave.
2. *Fred* came.	Who came was Fred.
3. Pete has *a tree house*.	What Pete has is a tree house.
4. Pete went *to buy bread*.	Why Pete went was to buy bread.
5. The dog chewed *the shoe*.	What the dog chewed was the shoe.

Perform *it* replacement and clause movement on the following sentences:

1. What he wants is this.	It is this that he wants.
2. Where it lives is in a nest.	It is in a nest that it lives.
3. Who Joe likes is a secret.	It is a secret who Joe likes.
4. Why he came was to pick peaches.	It was to pick peaches that he came.

ADVERBIAL CLAUSES AND
CONJUNCTIVE ADVERBS

T HE SYNTACTIC COMPLEXITY of the adverbial clauses varies
from simple to quite complex. The more complex forms
will receive further consideration in the chapters on comparative
constructions and on cause and effect. The conjunctive adverbs
are not similar syntactically to the adverbial clauses. However,
there are parallels between them in terms of the meaning relationships which both forms permit.

ADVERBIAL CLAUSES

Adverbial clauses are introduced by such words as *because,
when, although, if, unless, until, after,* etc. Most of them are
transformationally formed simply by placing one of the appropriate introductory words in front of a sentence. These introductory
words, sometimes called subordinating conjunctions, each have
a specific meaning. This meaning determines the logical relationship which the adverbial clause has with the main sentence
to which it has been joined. These meanings and logical relationships are often classified as cause, condition, concession, comparison, location, manner, purpose and time.

Some of the adverbial clauses are moveable. This movement,
though, is usually restricted to pre- and postmain sentence positions:

1. *When Fred bought the car,* he sold his bike.
2. Joe called Fred *when he was ready to go.*
3. *If you want a pickle,* raise your hand.

When adverbial clauses appear at the beginning of a sentence they are often marked by a comma.

Clauses of place or location are sometimes more restricted in movement:

4. Joe parked the car *where Fred wanted it.*
5. He put the cookies *where everyone could reach them.*
6. Pete lives *where he works.*

Examples 4 and 5 have transitive main verbs which very naturally take adverb of place complements. The verb *put* actually requires an adverb of place as a complement. Sentence 6 has an intransitive verb which generally requires an adverb of place. In sentences such as these, the normal position for the location clause is at the end of the sentence.

Clauses of manner are most normally placed after the verb:

7. He ran *as if a lion were chasing him.*
8. The car looked *as though it had been wrecked.*

Clauses indicating result or comparison have a fixed position because they have a point of connection with the main sentence. This point of connection is an adjective, an adverb or a noun phrase which is a part of the main sentence.

9. Fred is *as* tall *as Pete is.* (adjective)
10. Joe walked *so* quickly *that he caught up with Jill.* (adverb)
11. Jill has *as much* money *as April spent.* (noun)

The introductory elements in these clauses come in pairs such as *er than, as . . . as, so . . . that.* The first member of the pair will either precede or affix to the connecting word in the main sentence. The second member of the pair will precede the adverbial clause.

Often the sequence subject, tense and *be* is deleted from adverbial clauses. This deletion occurs when the subject of the clause is the same as the clause of the main sentence:

12. *When the dog was* (becomes) *When happy,* the dog
    happy, the dog   wagged its tail.
    wagged its tail.
13. *If you are working* (becomes) *If working in the library,*
    in the library, be   be quiet.
    quiet.

14. *Although Joe was big*   *Although big for his age,*
    for his age, he couldn't   he couldn't ride the bike.
    ride the bike.

Some conditional clauses can be formed without the subordinating conjunction *if*. In such instances, the subject and auxiliary transpose as in a yes/no question:

15. *If I had known,* I   [or]   *Had I known,* I would
    would have helped.   have helped.
16. *If you were going,*   [or]   *Were you going,* then we
    then we would go.   would go.

For a conditional clause to be formed in this manner requires a complex auxiliary in the conditional sentence. Simple past or present tense forms of transitive or intransitive verbs cannot form conditional clauses in this way. They must have the *if* form.

CONJUNCTIVE ADVERBS

Conjunctive adverbs seem parallel to the subordinating conjunction in some meaning relationships. Conjunctive adverbs include words such as *therefore, however, consequently, nevertheless, moreover,* etc. These words relate the sentence in which they appear to a previous sentence or sentences. Conjunctive adverbs may be placed at the beginning, middle or end of the sentence without changing meaning:

1. Joe was very tired; *nevertheless,* he continued on.
2. It began to rain; the game *consequently* was stopped.
3. We liked the car; we did not buy it, *however.*

These examples show the sentences punctuated with semicolons. However, sentences joined by conjunctive adverbs may be punctuated with periods or colons.

CONCLUSION

The adverbial clauses have the structural forms which permit the communication of the more complex concepts and reasoning. Clauses of cause, reason, condition or concession can enter the language repertoire of a child only when he has arrived at that state of cognitive maturation and has had sufficient experience. This cognitive level of maturation is the primary determinant for ordering the learning of some of the specific logical forms of adverbial clauses. The syntactic form which is basic to most of them can be learned fairly early if they are conceptually simple forms such as location.

ADVERBS

I N PREVIOUS CHAPTERS adverbials in the forms of clauses and phrases have been discussed. The clauses were related to sentences by subordinating conjunctions in a variety of logical relationships such as cause, condition, time, etc. Prepositional phrases which indicate the adverbial function of location, time and manner were illustrated. In addition to prepositional phrases which indicate time and location, single word forms can be used with the same effect. One-word adverbs of time include *now, then, already, yesterday, tomorrow,* etc. The single-word adverbs of place include *here, there* and *near.* In the last chapter the conjunctive adverbs (therefore, however, moreover, etc.) were discussed. These were single word forms, but they had a primary syntactic function of joining sentences in certain logical relationships.

The adverbs under consideration in this chapter are primarily the single word forms. However, adverbs are not a homogenous class of words which operate with syntactic regularity and with uniformity of meaning. Most adverbs are derived from adjectives, nouns or verbs and as a consequence retain the characteristics of their respective origins. Also, they may appear in an almost bewildering variety of sentence positions.

ADVERBS OF MANNER

Most adverbs originate from other word forms. Their transformation to adverbs takes more or less circuitous routes. The manner adverbs are the most varied in form and function.

Manner adverbs may readily appear with transitive and intransitive verbs:

1. He opened the box *quickly*.   (transitive)
2. He drove *carefully*.   (intransitive)

With more restrictions, they can occur with verbs like *become, seem* or *appear:*

3. He would become active *unwillingly*.
4. They looked angry *playfully*.

SOURCES. A good many nouns can become adverbs of manner. However, the first step in this process is the change to an adjective by adding an appropriate adjectival suffix. These suffixes include *full, less, ish, al, ous, ic* and *ate*. After the adjective suffix is added, a form of the adverb suffix *ly* is added. This process accounts for such adverbial forms as *gracefully, emotionally, needlessly, foolishly,* etc.

Adverbs of manner can be derived from various verbs. The derivation here again will require the change to an adjective by means of an appropriate affix and then to the adverb by the addition of *ly*. The adjective-forming suffixes used with verbs include *ent, ant, ive* and *able*. Adverbs formed in this manner are *confidently, pleasantly, selectively* and *agreeably*. Present and past participial forms of some verbs may form adverbs by simply adding the *ly* suffix. Included in this group are *decidedly, hurriedly, charmingly* and *lovingly*.

Adjectives may directly form adverbs of manner by the addition of the *ly* suffix. Here we have such words as *adequately, intelligently, clearly, politely, sadly,* etc. Some adjectives form adverbs with no suffix necessary. Such adjectives or adverbs include *bright, deep, hard, fast, straight,* etc.

A number of prepositional phrases can be used to introduce adverbs of manner. Some prepositions are more productive in this regard than are others. The preposition *by* is used to introduce several forms. It can introduce a phrase containing nominalized sentences as in the following examples:

1. Joe earned the money *by delivering papers*.
2. The bird got the worm *by rising early*.

Another common form indicates the measure by which things are sold:

3. Cloth is sold *by the yard.*
4. Eggs are sold *by the dozen.*

By is also used in other complex prepositional phrase forms such as *by means of*—and *by virtue of* —.

The preposition *in* will introduce quite a number of idiomatic adverbs of manner such as *in a hurry, in a pinch, in vain, in short,* etc. *In* will also introduce the prepositional phrase forms *in this way* and *in that way.* This form may be expanded to include an adjective such as *in a humorous way, in a happy way, in an abrupt way,* etc. The word *manner* is interchangeable with *way* in these forms.

The preposition *with* is used to introduce manner adverbials of several types including some like

5. Jill came *with Fred.*
6. The boy opened the bank *with a hammer.*
7. The children laughed *with enthusiasm.*

There are a number of proforms which may be used for adverbs of manner. These are *somehow, anyhow, someway* and *anyway.* Possibly included are the phrases which were mentioned earlier *(in) this way* and *(in) that way,* also the words *thus* and *so* function as proform replacements for adverbs of manner.

POSITION. The examples of adverbs of manner which have been presented so far have appeared at the end of sentences. However, they may appear just before the verbs and at the beginning of sentences as well. Consider these examples with the alternate positions:

9. He *quickly* opened the box.
10. *Carefully* Fred drove home.
11. Jill, *by saving her money,* bought a horse.

Manner adverbs are a very diverse group, however they have one fundamentally unifying characteristic. This characteristic is that they all may be replaced by the interrogative word *how* in the formation of questions. The following examples are question transformations of examples 9, 10 and 11:

12. How did he open the box?

13. How did Fred drive home?
14. How did Jill buy a horse?

ADVERBS OF FREQUENCY

The adverbs of frequency have a certain amount of mobility as do the manner adverbs. However, the most natural place for adverbs of frequency is before the verb. The adverbs of frequency which have the most freedom of movement include *frequently, occasionally* and *sometimes.*

Adverbs of frequency describe many levels of frequency from *always* to *never.* Some of the common forms in addition to the ones mentioned include *often, regularly, once in a while, usually,* etc.

The words *once* and *twice* are used in this adverbial form. After *twice* the usual procedure is to form a noun phrase of the form cardinal number plus the word *times.* This procedure forms noun phrases such as *three times, four times,* etc.

Other noun phrases can be used with *every* and *each* as in *everyday, every other day, each Christmas,* etc.

One prepositional phrase form introduced by *on* is quite commonly used with days of the week as an adverb of frequency. Such phrases include *on Mondays, on Fridays.*

The suffix *ly* may be added to certain nouns that have a time feature to produce adverbs of frequency. These include *weekly, monthly, daily, hourly,* etc.

The interrogative form *how often* is used in the formation of questions concerning adverbs of frequency:

1. How often do you drive?
2. How often is your doctor in his office?

Unlike adverbs of manner, adverbs of frequency may occur with *be:*

3. Joe is *often* happy.
4. Fred is at school *occasionally.*

ADVERBS OF SEQUENCE

Some adverbs indicate organizational sequence. *Then* is commonly used to indicate sequence in time. Ordinals such as *first, second, third* and *next* may be used in this fashion both by themselves and in prepositional phrases introduced by *in*.

1. *First,* he bought a Ford; and *second,* he bought a Peugeot.
2. *In the first place,* she was right.

NEGATIVE ADVERBS

Some adverbs have negative connotations. Some such as *never* are clearly negative while *seldom* and *rarely* are not distinctly so.

When these adverbs appear in the initial part of a sentence, they require a change in word order which is similar to that of yes/no questions:

1. *Never* have I seen a rhino.
2. *Rarely* did Joe miss recess.
3. *Seldom* was the train on time.

Other adverbs in this class are *scarcely, hardly, barely,* etc.

ADVERBS OF EXTENT

This group of adverbs will appear before adjectives. These adverbs are frequently made from adjectives with the *ly* suffix. The group includes forms as in

1. He felt *awfully* hungry.
2. He was *keenly* aware of the opportunity.
3. They were *entirely* wrong.
4. The housing was *grossly* inadequate.

This group of adverbs includes *relatively, absolutely, actually, badly, highly, remarkably,* etc.

An overlapping set of adverbs which also modify adjectives is called intensifiers. This set includes *very, quite, extremely, so* and *too*. When *so* and *too* are used in this manner, they require stress which is not obligatory for the other intensifiers:

5. Joe was *very* tired.
6. Jill was *quite* happy.
7. His car was *too* long.
8. The birds were *so* loud.

Intensifiers may also be used to modify some adverbs of frequency:

9. They came *quite* frequently.
10. He came *very* often.

SENTENCE ADVERBIALS

Sentence adverbials are divided into two classes (Schreiber, 1971). The first class is labeled as modal adverbs. This class includes *apparently, certainly, clearly, obviously, probably,* etc. The second class is called evaluative adverbs. This class includes *astonishingly, fortunately, interestingly, luckily, oddly, strangely, unfortunately,* etc. Modal adverbs suggest a degree of likelihood while evaluative adverbs offer judgment about something assumed to be true.

Most sentence adverbs are produced from adjectives by the addition of the *ly* suffix. The exceptions are words like *perhaps* and *indeed.* A good many words used as sentence adverbs may also be used as adverbs of manner. It is this overlap which may cause some difficulty. The primary distinction between sentence adverbs and adverbs of manner is that the *how* question form cannot be used with sentence adverbs. Sentence adverbs may occupy the pre- and postsentence positions as do the manner adverbs. The correct interpretation, then, requires the appropriate use of context to identify the intended meaning. Consider the interpretations of the following sentences:

1. *Clearly* Joe answered the question.
2. Pete came to school *oddly.*

If the writer's or speaker's intent has to do with likelihood or truth of the sentence, then they are sentence adverbs and no *how* question may be directed to the adverb. If, however, the intent has to do with the way or manner in which things were conducted, then these words are manner adverbs and the *how* question is appropriately directed to the adverbs. It might be added that sentence adverbs are often marked by commas.

Some sentence adverbs need to be coupled with *enough* to clearly distinguish them from adverbs of manner. This group includes *astonishingly, curiously, remarkably, surprisingly, oddly, strangely,* etc. Some examples are

3. *Strangely enough,* Joe answered the question.
4. *Oddly enough,* Pete came to school.

This group is semantically characterized by a degree of incredulity, especially when *enough* is used with the adverbs:

ALMOST, NEARLY AND HARDLY

This set of adverbs appears with some noun phrases and with some verbs. *How* questions are not directed to these adverbs. *Almost* and *nearly* appear with noun phrases that have determiner structures such as *none of* and *all of:*

1. *Almost* none of the plants were wilted.
2. *Nearly* all of the children were on time.
3. *Almost* all of the plants bloomed.

Hardly, as well as the more widely used adverbs *scarcely* and *barely,* may appear with noun phrases which have *any* in their determiner.

4. *Hardly* any of the plants were wilted.
5. *Scarcely* any of the children came to the party.

This set of adverbs appears with verbs in sentences such as

6. He *almost* dropped the box.
7. Fred *nearly* fell asleep.
8. He *barely* escaped.

JUST, EVEN, ONLY

These three adverbs have the greatest flexibility in terms of the various sentence positions in which they may appear. They may appear before noun phrases:

1. He ate *just* one doughnut.
2. *Only* Jill had a cold.
3. They didn't have *even* one car.

Of the three words, *only* alone will appear in a noun modifier position. This is probably because *even* and *just* also have adjective forms which mean *level* and *fair* respectively. If *even* and *just* appear in noun modifier positions, then they are interpreted as adjectives:

1. We have the *only* python on the block.
2. He is a *just* man. (adjective)
3. This isn't an *even* seam. (adjective)

Just, even and *only* are often used before the subordinating conjunction which introduces adverbial clauses:

4. They got on the train *just* as it was leaving.
5. They will come *even* if you don't want them.
6. He will go to sleep *only* when it is dark.

Just, even and *only* may be used with prepositional phrases.

7. They feed *just* at night.
8. She works *only* on foreign cars.
9. He gave a dime *even* to Fred.

Of the three, just *only* will appear following the prepositional phrases:

10. They feed at night *only*.
11. She works on foreign cars *only*.

The three words may appear before adverbs. In these cases the meaning seems about the same as if they appeared before the verb:

12. The car runs *just* adequately.
13. The car doesn't run *even* poorly.
14. *Just* then the train moved.

When *only* is used with an adverb at the beginning of a sentence, then that sentence will take the form of a yes/no question:

15. *Only* then did the grain move.
16. *Only* now can he stand on his head.

All three words operate freely with the various comparative constructions:

17. She is *just* as tall as April.
18. I can run *even* faster than Fred.
19. Pete has *only* as much money as Jill.

In addition to the functions illustrated above, the word *just* has a number of figurative or idiomatic uses as well. These include forms such as:

20. *Just* where do you think you're going?
21. *Just* you wait!
22. He might *just* as well go.

CONCLUSION

The various forms and functions of adverbs all pose problems for the language-handicapped child. Additionally, the derivation of many of the adverbs from nouns, adjectives or verbs may require attention in order to comprehend characteristics which are due to their respective points of origin. Also, potential problems are the variety of positions which they may hold and the yes/no word order changes that are functions of some adverb forms.

More detailed discussions of adverbs are available in papers by Nilsen (1972) and Schrieber (1971). A more detailed consideration of *just, even* and *only* is provided by Hargis (1975a).

COMPARATIVE CONSTRUCTIONS

COMPARATIVE CONSTRUCTIONS PROVIDE a basic part of the syntactic framework for the communication of some very important cognitive processes. These processes were described by Piaget as seriation and conservation. Seriation is the mental ability to order elements according to increasing or decreasing length, weight or volume. Conservation is the mental ability to realize that the amount or quantity of substances or matter stays the same even though its shape or position is changed. Arithmetic reasoning assumes these cognitive structures and expands into a variety of other cognitive areas. However, the comparative constructions are among the most common forms that indicate the type of mathematical operation to be performed (Hargis, 1975b).

In the chapter on adverbial clauses the comparatives were briefly mentioned. They were placed in a class of adverbial clauses which were linked with a word in the main sentence. These words are adjectives, nouns or adverbs. The conceptual basis for comparisons is equality or differences in those things or traits being compared.

AS ... AS

The as .... as comparative transformation joins sentences when the conceptual intent is the same level of equality. The word *as* precedes the linking word and the second *as* introduces the adverbial clause.

Adjectives may be compared:

   1. Jill is tall.

T-comparative   Jill is *as* tall *as* April
                                              (is) _____.

   April is tall.

Comparative constructions are subject to various deletions. The deletion is indicated by what elements in the adverbial clause are common to the main sentence. In example 1 notice that the word tall is deleted obligatorily. The deletion is indicated by the _____. Parenthesis around *is* indicates that it may optionally be deleted.

Adverbs may be compared:

   2. Fred left quickly.

T-comparative   Fred left *as* quickly *as* Joe
                                              (did) _____.

   Joe left quickly.

In example 2 the redundant verb *left* may be reduced to the verb proform *do. Do* used in this fashion will carry the indicator of tense and agreement which was formerly held by the verb. The second adverb is obligatorily deleted.

Count nouns may be compared:

   3. Joe has toys.

T-comparative   Jill has *as* many toys *as* April
                                              (has or does) _____.

   April has toys.

The as . . . as comparison of count nouns requires the introduction of the quantifier word *many*.

When noncount nouns are compared, the quantifier word used is *much:*

   4. Joe has milk.

T-comparative   Joe has *as much* milk *as*
                                              Pete (has or does) _____.

   Pete has milk.

The *as . . . as* comparative form also represents the syntactic form for multiplication. Consider these sentences.

5. Joe has *twice as much* money *as* Fred has.
6. Pete has *three times as many* marbles *as* Jill has.
7. Fred is *half as* tall *as* the tree.

In example 6 any number could be used, depending on what the multiplier is. In example 7 any fraction could be used.

When the compared adjectives are embedded in the noun modifier position of the main sentence rather than in a free position, as in example 1, an additional alteration is necessary:

8. Joe has a *nice* dog.

T-comparative	Joe has *as nice* a dog *as* Fred (has or does) _____.
Fred has a nice dog.	[or]
	Joe has a dog *as nice as* Fred (has or does) _____.

The embedded adjective must be removed with *as* to the pre or postnoun phrase position.

ER ... THAN, MORE ... THAN

The conceptual basis for this comparative transformation is inequality between the compared things.

Adjectives may be compared:

1. Jill is tall.

T-comparative	Jill is tall*er than* April (is) _____.
April is tall.	

The *er* is affixed to the first adjective and *than* introduces the adverbial clause.

When adverbs are compared, the form *more....than* is used.

2. Joe sings beautifully.

T-comparative	Joe sings *more* beautifully *than* Fred (does) _____.
Fred sings beautifully.	

More is used to introduce multisyllable adjectives as well as adverbs.

Count and noncount nouns are compared in the same way.

3. Jill has toys.

T-comparative

April has toys.

Jill has *more* toys *than* April (has) _____.

4. Joe has milk.

T-comparative

Pete has milk.

Joe has *more* milk *than* Pete (has or does) _____.

LESS ... THAN, FEWER ... THAN

Comparisons may be made in the diminutive direction. Adjectives and adverbs may be compared.

1. Mary is beautiful.

T-comparative

Alice is beautiful.

Mary is *less* beautiful *than* Alice (is) _____.

2. The lion roars loudly.

T-comparative

The tiger roars loudly.

The lion roars *more* loudly *than* the tiger (does) _____.

When count nouns are compared in this direction, the form *fewer.....than* is ordinarily used.

3. Jill has toys.

T-comparative

April has toys.

Jill has *fewer* toys *than* April (has or does) _____.

Noncount nouns are compared with *less....than*.

4. Joe has milk.

T-comparative

Fred has milk.

Joe has *less* milk *than* Fred (has or does) _____.

More....than and *less....than* may be used as adverbials if the compared adverb is sufficiently well understood.

5. Joe walks often.

T-comparative   Joe walks *more than* he runs.
Joe runs often.   [or]
                             Joe walks *more (often)* than
                             he runs.

BETTER THAN AND WORSE THAN

The adjectives *good* or *bad* and the adverbs *well* and *badly* may be compared. When they are, the comparative forms used are *better than* and *worse than,* respectively, for each word class.

THE SAME . . . AS, SAME AS AND DIFFERENT . . . THAN (FROM)

The *same. . . .as* and *same as* forms are used when identical things, characteristics, amounts or numbers are being compared:

1. Joe has a little juice.

T-comparative   Joe has the *same amount* of
                             juice *as* Fred (does) _____.
Fred has a little juice.

2. Joe has orange juice.

T-comparative   Joe has the *same kind* of
                             juice *as* Pete (does) _____.
Pete has orange juice.

The words that may appear between *same* and *as* are a general label for the class of things being compared. These words include *height, manner, way, style,* etc.

3. Fred goes in Fred's car.

T-comparative   Fred goes in *the same* car as
                             Pete (does) _____.
Pete goes in Fred's car.

4. Her name is Jones.

T-comparative   Her name is the *same as* your
                             name.
Your name is Jones.

When disparate characteristics are compared, then the *different . . . .than* or *different. . . .from* forms are used. Occasionally, when manner adverbs are the basis for comparison, the *ly* suffix will be attached to *different*. Otherwise, structurally, these have the same forms as do the *same. . . .as* or *same as:*

5. Her name is Jones

T-comparative　　　　　　　　　Her name is *different than* your (name) _____.

Your name is Smith.

NEGATIVE FORMS

The negative particles *not* or *no* may be used with some comparative forms Only *not* may be used with *as. . . .as* forms. Semantically, there are different purposes for *not* and for *no* when they are used with comparatives:

1. Joe is tall.

T-comparative　　　　　　　　　Joe is *not taller than* Pete (is) _____.

Pete is tall.　　　　　　　　　　　[or]

Joe is no taller than Pete (is) _____.

SUPERLATIVES AND COMPARATIVES

Some comparative forms may appear as prearticles. However, the primary form for superlative constructions is the prearticle form. The syntactic frame *the. . . .er* is used for comparatives, and the frame *the. . . .est* of it used for the superlative. The comparative prearticle indicates the selection of one from a compared set of two. The superlative prearticle indicates the selection of one from a compared set of more than two.

1. Joe is *the taller of* the (two) boys.
2. Pete is *the tallest of* the (five) girls.

The *est* affix often is simply added to adjectives to form this frame, but there are other superlative words which may be used in this prearticle frame. These include *least, most, best* and *worst*. These forms may undergo reductions similar to those of other noun phrases with prearticles.

PROBLEMS IN COMPARATIVE FORMS

Redundant or duplicate elements are often obligatorily deleted or reduced as a result of comparative transformations. Other elements are optionally deleted. This reduction of information will require the greatest use of context and the familiarity with the base sentences from which the comparative form was produced. The following sentence shows the reduction to only one word from the original base sentence:

1. The bush is wider than _____ _____ tall.

The sentence appears short and simple, but it requires considerable use of syntactic context to fill in the reduced gaps produced in this comparative transformation.

Some sentences may become ambiguous as the result of reduction:

2. Jill likes Fred as much as April.

The following examples illustrate the possible source sentences which could be the basis for sentence 2:

3. Jill likes Fred.

T-comparative　　　　　　　　Jill likes Fred as much as
　　　　　　　　　　　　　　　(she likes) April.

　　Jill likes April.
4. Jill likes Fred

T-comparative　　　　　　　　Jill likes Fred as much as
　　　　　　　　　　　　　　　April (likes Fred).

　　April likes Fred.

Comparative forms themselves may undergo comparative transformations. These result in exceedingly complex forms. Consider the following examples which contain three comparative transformations:

5. Jill has money.

T-comparative　　　　　　　　Jill has *more* money *than*
　　　　　　　　　　　　　　　April _____ _____.

　　April has money.
6. Fred has money.

T-comparative　　　　　　　　Fred has *more* money *than*
　　　　　　　　　　　　　　　Pete _____ _____.

　　Pete has money.

Then, by comparing the results of 5 and 6,

7. Jill has *more* money
   than April _____ _____.

T-comparative   Jill has *as much more* money
                                         than April _____ _____ *as* Fred
                                         has *more* money than Pete _____
                                         _____.

Fred has more money
than Pete _____ _____.

For those interested in more detailed or theoretical considerations of aspects of comparative constructions, papers by Lees (1961) and Bresnan (1973, 1975) provide substantial information.

EXERCISES

Identify the sentences which comprise the following comparative constructions:

	Answers
1. Joe runs faster than Fred	a. Joe runs fast.
	b. Fred runs fast.
2. Zeke has fewer problems than Joe.	a. Zeke has problems.
	b. Joe has problems.
3. He is as tall as she.	a. He is tall.
	b. She is tall.
4. He sings as badly as he plays.	He sings badly.
	b. He plays badly
5. The boy swims as poorly as he runs well.	a. The boy swims poorly.
	b. The boy runs well.

PARTICIPIAL AND ABSOLUTE PHRASES

THE TWO STRUCTURES under consideration in this chapter have some surface resemblances. They both originate from sentences. However, their source and the logical relationships that they hold with the sentences to which they are combined are different.

PARTICIPIAL PHRASES

In Chapter 15 some participial phrases were discussed that were complements of transitive verbs. The participial phrases in this chapter are related to nonrestrictive relative clauses. Their function is like that of appositives.

1. *Patting the puppy's head,* he told it to sit.
2. *Having done well on the test,* Joe got an A in the course.
3. *Dropped from the second floor,* the ball bounced.
4. *Forgotten by the children,* the dog wandered away.

The subject of the sentence from which these phrases originated is the same as the subject of the main sentence. Like relative clauses and appositives, they could follow the subject of the main sentence, but, unlike other appositive forms, only those which contain either the present or past participle will ordinarily shift to the beginning of the sentence. These structures may also appear at the end of the main sentence as well. Wherever the participial phrase appears it will be set off by commas to indicate the pauses which separate it from the main sentence.

If the subject of the main sentence is a personal pronoun, the shift to the beginning of the sentence seems to be more desirable.

5. *Sliding into the base,* he beat the ball.

The present participle affix (ing) replaces tense in the auxiliary of the sentences which are transformed into participial phrases. This was illustrated in examples 1, 2 and 5. Traditional modals cannot appear in participial phrases since they cannot accept the *ing* affix. The past participle affix will appear in the participial phrase when the sentence from which it is derived is passive. This is illustrated by examples 3 and 4.

The so-called dangling participle occurs when the subject of the participial phrase is not identified by the main sentence. This may happen when the main sentence is passive.

6. *Walking out of sight,* Fred was forgotten by Joe. The problem in example 6 is whether the subject of the participial phrase is *Fred* or *Joe.* Other such problems occur when the subjects are not shared at all.

ABSOLUTE PHRASES

The constructions under consideration here have traditionally been called nominative absolutes. Unlike the participial phrases, they do not share subjects with the main sentence. Consequently, the subject of the absolute phrase is retained:

1 *The game having ended,* the crowd left the ball park.
2. *Their feet dangling in the water,* the children fished all afternoon.
3. We will have the party outdoors, *weather permitting.*
4. *Their mittens lost,* the children cried.
5. *The meal on the table,* the cook took a break.
6. *The children home from school,* the dog started barking.

Absolute phrases take two forms. The tense may be replaced by the *ing* affix as in examples 1, 2 and 3, or *tense* and *be* may be deleted from the auxiliary as in 4, 5 and 6. These phrases appear at either end of the main sentence.

Absolute constructions express many of the same relationships that adverbial clauses do. Possibly absolute phrases are reduced forms of adverbial clauses. Examples 1 through 6 have meanings which are more directly expressed by adverbial clauses. The relationships expressed in these examples are respectively cause, attendant circumstances, condition, cause, time and cause.

CONCLUSION

Participial and absolute phrases are reduced forms of other syntactic structures. These structures have more obvious surface clues as to their relationship to main sentences than do the phrases. In other words, this reduction gives less direct indication of meaning relationships. This causes the consequent difficulty in dealing with participial and absolute forms.

Since these structures are reductions of relative or adverbial clauses, the order for teaching them should be from the clause to the phrase forms. Comprehension of the phrase forms can only grow from mastery of the clause forms.

EXERCISES

Identify the sentences underlying the following participial and absolute phrases:

1. Having completed his work, Joe left.

    Joe had completed his work.

2. A tree having fallen across the road, traffic was backed up for miles.

    A tree had fallen across the road.

3. The children in bed, father turned off the lights.

    The children were in bed.

4. The trees stirred in the wind, their leaves a bright yellow.

    Their leaves were a bright yellow.

5. Thinking about the party, Joe excitedly ran home.

    Joe thought about the party.

6. Thrown in the lake two years before, the bottle washed up at the same spot on the beach.

    The bottle was thrown in the lake two years before.

CAUSE AND EFFECT

I N THE CHAPTER on comparative constructions, the content was related to areas of cognitive development in childhood. This chapter contains a composite of varied syntactic structures which represent an area of cognitive development in children. Many of the structures have been introduced in previous chapters, but the purpose here is to organize all of the structures which serve this cognitively and linguistically difficult area.

The area of cognitive development has to do with the awareness of causality or cause and effect relationships. The syntactic structures covered are quite varied. Cause and effect reasoning itself is at least as varied as the syntactic structures which represent it in our language. Some structures are used for the representation of direct cause and effect relationships. Others represent only sufficiency for a causal relationship. Still others indicate negative causal relationships. Also, some structures move from causality into the area of purpose. In some structures the causal component is emphasized while in others the effect or consequence receives emphasis.

WHY, WHAT . . . FOR, AND HOW COME

The *wh* questions used to interrogate these structures are the *why, what. . . .for* and *how come* questions. These questions are among the most difficult. This is true because of the varied and complex structures, both cognitively and linguistically, which they interrogate (Hargis, 1972, 1975c). Regardless of the structural form the sentence takes, the interrogative word or words will replace the causal component. Given the cause and effect sentence il-

174

lustrated in example 1, the subsequent examples illustrate the question forms used to interrogate it.

1. Joe went to bed because he was sleepy.
2. Why did Joe go to bed?
3. What did Joe go to bed for?
4. How come Joe went to bed?

Examples 2, 3 and 4 are the three question forms which may be directed to the cause and effect relationship expressed in sentence 1. The three question forms seem essentially synonymous even if structurally different. Zwickey (1972) discusses in detail the three question forms. He also comments on the interesting lack of a yes/no question component in the *how come* question forms.

SO THAT

So that introduces a causal abverbial clause in sentences such as

1. Mary saved her money *so that she could buy a new bike.*
2. Fred got up early *so that he could get to school on time.*

The word *that* may be deleted with no alteration in meaning. The *so* may be replacd by the words *in order.* In this instance the *that* is not deletable. There is one restriction on the causal sentences used in this class. These sentences appear to require a modal form in their auxiliaries.

SO ... THAT

In this class the words *so. . . .that* link two sentences in the cause and effect relationship. The basis, or linking point, for this relationship is an adjective, an adverb or a noun phrase. The *so* precedes the adjective, adverb or noun phrase and the *that* introduces the effect sentence.

1. Fred was *so* sleepy *that he went to bed.*
2. Joe was *so* tall *that he could reach the shelf.*
3. Pete came *so* often *that he knew everyone.*
4. Joe had *so* many marbles *that he gave some to Fred.*
5. Joe got a raise *so* small *that he was unhappy.*

The *that* is readily deleted from this construction. When a linking adjective appears in the noun modifier position, *so* plus the adjective must be moved to either a pre- or postnoun phrase position. In example 5 it holds the postnoun phrase position. The prenoun phrase position for the same sentence is illustrated in example 6:

6. Joe got *so* small a raise *that he was unhappy.*

There are rules governing the movement of *so* plus the adjective. If the noun phrase containing the adjective has the article *a(n)* or *some, so* plus the adjective may move to either the pre- or postnoun phrase position. If the noun phrase has a definite article or the zero article, then *so* plus the adjective will appear only in the postnoun phrase position.

SUCH ... THAT

This structure links sentences on the basis of noun phrases. *Such* may either precede or follow the noun phrase while *that* will introduce the effect clause.

1. He was *such* a good student *(that) he got all A's.*

That is deletable in structures where *such* precedes the noun phrase.

THAT

In this class of cause and effect sentences *that* introduces the causal clause.

1. Jill was happy *that she got a puppy.*
2. Fred seemed sad *that he graduated.*

That is used in cause and effect structures in rather restricted circumstances. The clause which expresses the effect must contain a copulative verb form followed by adjectives indicating emotion.

SO

Here, *so* introduces the clause which expresses effect or consequence.

1. The sun went down *so the birds stopped singing.*
2. It was a holiday *so the school was empty.*

The three different uses for *so* in cause and effect sentences may well be a source of difficulty. This difficulty may be further compounded by the additional uses of *so* as an intensifier and in affirmation.

Conjunctive adverbs including *therefore, consequently, as a result* and *as a consequence* have essentially the same meaning as *so*. They will appear with or within the effect or consequence clause, but they have the same mobility features as do all of the conjunctive adverbs.

BECAUSE, SINCE, AS

Because introduces causal clauses. *Since* and *as* may perform in essentially the same manner. *For* is also used, but much more rarely today to introduce causal clauses of the same type. *Because* may ordinarily be substituted for the other three forms with no change in meaning:

1. Fred went home *because he was tired.*
2. Jill has been sad *since April left.*
3. Helen left *as Joe arrived.*

There is possible ambiguity with *since* and *as* in sentences 2 and 3. Both *since* and *as* are used to introduce time clauses. The determination between time and cause produces the ambiguity. Perhaps the double connotation which *since* and *as* has caused their selection over *because* on certain occasions.

BECAUSE OF, DUE TO, ON ACCOUNT OF

Because of introduces a nominalized causal sentence. *Due to* and *on account of* perform similarly to *because of:*

1. Joe got an A *because of his hard work.*
2. *Due to heavy rain,* the streets were flooded.

These phrase forms are probably reductions of adverbial clauses which were introduced by *because.*

AS A RESULT OF, AS A CONSEQUENCE OF

As a result of and *as a consequence of* also introduce nominalized causal sentences. However, conceptually they are related to the *so* class where effect clauses are introduced and emphasized.

1. Joe was late to school *as a consequence of sleeping late.*
2. Pete lost three pounds *as a result of the flu.*

FROM

The prepositional phrase introduced by *from* can indicate causality. *Due to* and *because of* may be substituted for *from* when causality is indicated. A potential difficulty with this form is the fact that *from* more ordinarily has a directional or motion connotation which may interfere with the appropriate interpretation:

1. Joe's hands turned blue *from the cold.*
2. The dog died *from old age.*

OUT OF

This structure also has a more usual directional meaning which may cause difficulty. *Because of* may be substituted for it when causality is indicated. When *out of* is used to indicate causal relationships, it appears to be restricted to those which are emotional in nature:

1. He cried *out of frustration.*
2. She left *out of anger.*

FOR

The prepositional phrase introduced by the preposition *for* may indicate causality. The nominal form which follows *for* may be a noun phrase or a nominalized sentence. *For* structures cover the spectrum from purpose to cause. The *what. . . .for* question form is used interchangeably with *why.* When cause is implied the *what. . . .for* question must be used:

1. Joe got an electric car *for driving to work.*
2. He worked hard *for his club.*
3. She thanked the boy *for helping her.*
4. The book is *for you.*

Example 4 illustrates only purpose, while in example 2 either purpose or cause might be intended.

FOR ... TO

Sentences which have undergone the for/to transformation are frequently used to indicate causality:

1. We bought the bike *for the children to ride.*
2. The children took the animals to the pond *for them to get a drink.*
3. Joe goes to school *to play basketball.*

For plus the subject of the transformed sentence may be deleted when the subject is redundant, as in example 3.

TOO ... FOR ... TO

In this class of sentences, a negative causal relationship is produced. *Too* operates in an intensifier position within the causal clause which is followed by a sentence nominalized by the for/to transformation. The for/to structure indicates the *effect* structure in this sentence class:

1. The shelf was *too* high *for him to reach.*
2. The food was *too* hot *for Joe to eat.*
3. The car was *too* great a bargain *for him not to buy it.*

The sentences underlying the for/to transformation in examples 1 and 2 are negative, even though there is no surface indication of this fact. However, in example 3, the underlying sentence is positive even though the surface structure shows the negative particle. This phenomena makes these structures exceedingly difficult. The *so. . . .that* form can be used essentially synonymously without the extra difficulties this form holds. The presentation of this structure should follow mastery of the *so. . . .that* form.

The movement of adjectives embedded in noun modifier positions is the same as for *so. . . .that.* In example 3 *too* plus the adjective is moved to the prenoun phrase position.

ENOUGH ... FOR ... TO

This form is syntactically similar to the *too. . . .for. . . .to* form. However, in this case the relationship expressed is sufficient for a cause and effect relationship:

1. The girl saved *enough* money *to buy a bike.*
2. Joe picked *enough* apples *for them to eat.*
3. The ladder was long *enough to reach the roof.*
4. The fruit was ripe *enough for them to pick.*
5. He came often *enough to meet everyone.*
6. It was a stick long *enough to reach the apples.*

Enough may be used with nouns as in examples 1 and 2. If they are used with an adjective or adverbs, *enough* will follow the adjective or adverb as in examples 3, 4 and 5. If the adjective modifies a noun, then it will follow the noun phrase as in example 6.

COINCIDENTAL AND TEMPORAL RELATIONSHIPS

Syntactic structures which suggest co-occurrence in time may be used to indicate cause and effect relationships:

1. He gets sleepy *when he stays up late.*
2. He was hungry *when he woke up.*
3. Jill was happy *while she was in school.*
4. Joe cooked supper *while he watched television.*

Sentences 1 and 3 are more easily interpreted as cause and effect relationships. However, in sentences 2 and 4 this relationship is quite unlikely.

CONCLUSION

Cause and effect relationships may be developed in more complex ways than in single sentences. Causality may require much more than single phrases or clauses. Paragraphs, chapters or books are used to develop the relationship, but the essential cognitive and linguistic features of cause and effect relationships must be mastered first at the sentence level.

CONJUNCTIONS

T HE PRIMARY PURPOSE of conjunctions is in joining sentences. Conceptually, the meaning which results from joining sentences by conjunction transformations is only a modest addition to the meaning held by the sentences used independently. The great difficulty with conjoined forms results from the reduction and alteration that may occur when sentences undergo conjunction transformations.

COORDINATING CONJUNCTIONS

Coordinating conjunctions include *and, or* and *but*. The meaning relationship imposed between two sentences conjoined by these three forms is said to be additive, alternative and adversative, respectively.

AND. The most commonly used form is *and*. It also has the most variety in range of conjoined forms which can be produced between two sentences. The logical focus in two conjoined sentences is on the nonidentical parts of the two sentences. These parts or structures are called conjuncts. Noun phrases, verbs, verb phrases, auxiliary parts, relative clauses, adverbs, adverbial clauses, nominalized sentences—virtually all sentence parts or sentences may be conjuncts. The sentence parts which are identical to one another determine the nature of the reduction in the conjoined sentences. The type of conjuncts in the two sentences will determine the remainder of alterations which may occur as a result of the conjunction transformation.

If two sentences which have no identical parts are to be conjoined, then the entire sentences are conjuncts, and nothing may be reduced or altered as a result of the conjunction transformation. The conjunction *and* will simply be placed between the two sentences. In print a comma will precede this *and:*

1. *Jill* bought a dog.

T-conj.   Jill bought a dog, and April
                                   found a cat.

   April found a cat.

When two conjoined sentences have identical subject noun phrases, the second noun phrase may be deleted or reduced to a pronoun:

2. *Jill* bought a dog.

T-conj.   Jill bought a dog, and she
   Jill found a cat.   found a cat.

                                   [or]
                                   Jill bought a dog and found a
                                   cat.

When any element is deleted from the second conjoined sentence, the comma is not included before *and*.

When two conjoined sentences have identical noun phrase objects, the second noun phrase may be reduced to a pronoun but not deleted:

3. A boy saw *the dog*.

T-conj.   A boy saw the dog, and a girl
                                   heard it.

   A girl heard *the dog*.

If the object noun phrase of the first sentence is identical to the subject noun phrase of the second, the subject noun phrase may be reduced to a personal pronoun but not deleted:

4. A boy saw *the dog*.

T-conj.   A boy saw the dog and it ran
                                   away.

   The dog ran away.

The subject noun phrase of the first sentence may be identical to the object noun phrase of the second. In these instances the object noun phrase may be reduced to a personal pronoun but not deleted:

    5. *The boy* saw the bird.

T-conj.   The boy saw the bird and the
dog heard him.

    The dog heard *the boy*.

If the verbs of the two conjoined sentences are identical, the second verb is sometimes deleted:

    6. Joe *heard* the duck.

T-conj.   Joe heard the duck, and Fred
(heard) the dog.

    Fred *heard* the dog.

More than one component in the two sentences may be identical. If both the subject noun phrases and the object noun phrases of the two sentences are identical, then the second subject may be reduced to a pronoun or deleted. The second object may only be reduced to a pronoun. The words *too, also* or *as well* may be added at the end of these sentences:

    7. *The boy* saw *the bird*.

T-conj.   The boy saw the bird and (he)
heard it (too).

    The boy heard *the bird*.

If both the subjects and the verbs of the conjoined sentences are identical, then the reduction and deletion is the same as for subjects alone (example 2) and verbs alone (example 6). The words *too, also* and *as well* may be used with these sentences also:

    8. *Joe heard* the duck.

T-conj.   Joe heard the duck, and (he)
(heard) the dog (too).

    Joe heard the dog.   [or]

                               Joe heard the duck and also
the dog.

After the deletion in such forms the word *also* may appear immediately following *and* as in the last conjoined sentence in example 8.

If the entire verb phrase of each sentence is identical, the conjoined sentence may have a variety of forms. The entire verb phrase of the second sentence may be deleted and the subject conjunct moved to a position adjacent to the first subject conjunct. The verb may be replaced by the proform *do* followed by *too, also* or *as well*. Also the *do* proform may be transposed with the second subject in a form resembling a yes/no question. In this case *and so* is used to join the sentences:

9. Joe *heard the dog.*

T-conj.   Joe heard the dog and Fred
                                                 (heard the dog) (too).
          Fred *heard the dog.*   [or]
                                                 Joe and Fred heard the dog.
                                                           [or]
                                                 Joe heard the dog and Fred
                                                 did too.
                                                           [or]
                                                 Joe heard the dog and so did
                                                 Fred.

When both sentences such as those in example 9 are negative, several forms are possible. The word *either* may be used with the second sentence. The negative form *neither* will be used if the second sentence takes the form resembling a yes/no question. This structurally resembles the last sentence in example 9.

10. Joe *didn't hear the dog.*

T-conj.   Joe didn't hear the dog and
                                                 Fred didn't (hear the dog)
                                                 either.
          Fred *didn't hear the*   [or]
          dog.   Joe didn't hear the dog and
                                                 neither did Fred.

SERIES. More than one sentence may be conjoined. The resultant reduction to the syntactically similar conjuncts is called a series. Normally each conjunct is separated by a comma and the last two are joined by *and:*

11. *Fred saw* a lion.

T-conj.   Fred saw a lion, a tiger, and a
                                                 shark.
          Fred saw a tiger.

T-conj.

    Fred saw a shark.

NP AND NP. Some sentence environments require two or more noun phrases. In such environments *and* does not indicate that two sentences have been joined by the conjunction transformation:

12. Joe sat between Jill and April.
13. Combine ice cream and milk.
14. Joe and Fred sang a duet together.

The preposition like *between* (example 12) requires two nouns joined by *and* or a plural pronoun. Verbs such as *combine, mix, blend,* etc. (example 13) also require two or more nouns or a plural pronoun. Other environments which suggest *together with* (example 14) require two or more nouns joined by *and* or the plural pronoun.

NOR. When two negative sentences are conjoined, *nor* may be used to connect them. When *nor* is used the second sentence undergoes structural change which resembles yes/no questions. The use of *nor* removes the negative particle from the second sentence.

15. *Joe didn't see the truck.*

T-conj.   Joe didn't see the truck, nor
                              did Fred hear the plane.

    Fred didn't hear the
    plane.

OR. Conceptually the conjunction *or* is used to join alternative conjuncts. The deletion and reduction procedures are similar to those used with the conjunction *and.* Consider the following conjoined sentences containing *or:*

16. Fred will go to bed or father will be angry.
17. Joe likes to fish in streams or rivers.

BUT. The conjunction *but* joins conjuncts which have relationships that are unexpected or adversative:

18. Joe ran home.

T-conj.   Joe ran home, but Fred stayed.

    Fred stayed.

    19. Joe didn't go.

T-conj.   Joe didn't go, but Pete went.

                                      [or]

        Pete went.   Not Joe but Pete went.

    20. Fred can skate.

T-conj.   Fred can skate, but Joe can't (skate).

        Joe can't skate.   [or]

                          Fred can skate but not Joe.

Subject conjuncts may be joined by *but* only if the first sentence is negative. See the second conjoined sentence in example 19. In this case the negative particle *not* will precede the first subject while *but* appears between them.

Notice that if the negative is in the first sentence, the redundant elements are reduced from it (example 19). However, if the second sentence is negative, then it is reduced (example 20).

CORRELATIVE CONJUNCTIONS

Correlative conjunctions appear in pairs. Those under consideration here are *both . . . and, either . . . or* and *neither . . . nor.*

BOTH . . . AND. When the conjuncts of two conjoined sentences are both subjects, *both . . . and* may be used to join them. This transformation is quite likely an extension from sentences which have already been joined by *and*. The conjoined sentence in example,

    1. Joe left.

T-conj.   Joe left and Fred left.

        Fred left.   Joe and Fred left.

                          Both Joe and Fred left.

When noun phrase objects appear after identical verbs, the noun phrase objects may be joined by *both . . . and*. Again, this appears to be derived from sentences already conjoined by *and:*

2. Jill saw a rabbit.

T-conj.   Jill saw a rabbit and she saw
                                         a goat.

Jill saw a goat.   Jill saw a rabbit and a goat.
                                         Jill saw both a rabbit and a
                                         goat.

Other sentence parts may be joined by *both . . . and*. Consider
the following examples where adverbs and adjectives are conjoined:

3. Joe works both quickly and diligently.
4. The car is both fast and economical.

EITHER . . . OR. Sentences or sentence parts may be joined *by
either . . . or:*

5. Joe is in the yard.

T-conj.   Either Joe is in the yard, or
                                         he is in the basement.

Joe is in the   [or]
basement.   Joe is either in the yard or in
                                         the basement.
                                                   [or]
                                         Joe is in either the yard or
                                         the basement.

Either . . . or is quite closely related to the use of *or*. The word
either will simply precede the first conjunct.

NEITHER . . . NOR. This correlative conjunction is closely related to *nor*. Both conjoined sentences must be negative. The
word *neither is* placed before the first conjunct. This correlative
conjunction will not join sentence conjuncts. It will join all
sentence parts including subjects which *nor* cannot do alone.

6. Joe didn't have a dog.

T-conj.   Joe didn't have a dog nor did
                                         Fred (have a dog) .

Fred didn't have a   [or]
dog.   Neither Joe nor Fred have a
                                         dog.

Notice that the negative particle is omitted from both sentences when *neither . . . nor* is used.

CONCLUSION

Conjoined sentences may have several forms with the same meaning. This variety of forms is the source of confusion. Further, the deletion, reduction and structural alteration which conjoined sentences may incorporate cause difficulty far beyond the intrinsic conceptual difficulty that they are intended to convey.

Readers who are interested in research related to the comprehension and production of conjoined sentences are referred to articles by Wilbur, Montanelli and Quigley (1975).

EXERCISES

Identify the base sentences for the following conjoined sentences:

1. The boy had neither a dog nor a cat.
   a. The boy didn't have a dog.
   b. The boy didn't have a cat.

2. He didn't want to go, nor did he want to stay.
   a. He didn't want to go.
   b. He didn't want to stay.

3. Both Fred and Sam liked Sue.
   a. Fred liked Sue.
   b. Sam liked Sue.

4. Fred was in the eighth grade and so was Sam.
   a. Fred was in the eighth grade.
   b. Sam was in the eighth grade.

5. Sam was and is working at the station.
   a. Sam was working at the station.
   b. Sam is working at the station.

6. Joe couldn't and wouldn't drive a car.
   a. Joe couldn't drive a car.
   b. Joe wouldn't drive a car.

7. Not the boy but the girl won the prize.

   a. The boy didn't win the prize.

   b. The girl won the prize.

8. Joe but not Fred is twelve.

   a. Joe is twelve.

   b. Fred is not twelve.

9. Either Fred goes or Pete will.

   a. Fred will go.

   b. Pete will go.

EXCLAMATIONS AND COMMANDS

T HIS CHAPTER DEALS with two different sentence forms. The first, exclamations or exclamatory sentences, is produced by transformation. The second, commands or imperative sentences, can be listed among the simple sentence classes and is not the result of transformation.

EXCLAMATIONS

Exclamation sentences have a variety of forms. In print, the identifying feature of all forms is the exclamation point. Some forms are structurally altered by the exclamation transformation. This alteration resembles *wh* questions without the yes/no component. The focus of the exclamation transformation is on intensifiers:

1. You have a very pretty   What a pretty car you
               (by T-exclam)
    car.   have!
2. Joe is very tall.   How tall Joe is!
3. Jill works very quickly.   How quickly Jill works!

What and *how* are the two words that are used to replace intensifiers in this transformation. Notice that *what* replaces the intensifier which appears within the noun phrase in example 1. *How* replaces the intensifier which appears before free adjectives (example 2) and before adverbs (example 3). *What* or *how*, together with the noun phrase, adjective or adverb which the intensifier appeared in, is shifted to the front of the sentence. A variety of exclamatory words or phrases such as *oh, my, goodness gracious,* etc., may often precede *what* and *how* in exclamatory sentences.

In some instances the exclamation transformation may change the auxiliary structure of sentences. If the auxiliary of a sentence contains more than just tense, then the first element in the auxiliary will receive extra heavy stress. If only tense occurs with a main verb other than *be,* then *do* insertion is required and *do* receives the extra stress. *Do* insertion is illustrated in sentence 7 of the following examples:

4. The boy might go!
5. Jill is going!
6. She has gone!
7. He did go!

Occasionally exclamatory sentences will be formed by deleting the verb *be* and its auxiliary from a sentence and adding the exclamation point.

8. Fred a scholar!
9. April a football player!

On other occasions exclamatory structures may have even more reduced forms:

10. How wonderful!
11. What a beautiful tree!

These forms are reduced to the word or phrase which contained the intensifier that was replaced by *how* or *what.*

Normal question forms which are stated rhetorically may be used as exclamatory sentences. In print they will be punctuated with exclamation points rather than question marks.

COMMANDS

Commands or imperative sentences are most notable for the absence of a subject noun phrase in them. They are composed of such forms as

1. Get the paper for me.
2. Follow that cab.
3. Bring me a new pencil.

The underlying subject of all imperative sentences is *you*. No auxiliary element other than present tense is used in this sentence class. These sentence types can be changed to requests by adding the word *please*.

CONCLUSION

Conceptually, exclamatory sentences indicate things such as assertions of truth, surprise or incredulity. The problem of interpretation of these sentences may be resolved only by the effective use of whatever context is available.

The primary problem with the comprehension of imperative sentences is due to the lack of an apparent subject and that when this occurs the notion of command or request is intended.

DIRECT AND INDIRECT
DISCOURSE

D IRECT AND INDIRECT discourse forms are used to report conversation. Direct discourse provides a quotation or the
replica of what was said while the indirect discourse form provides a syntactically altered form from the actual structures which
were in fact expressed. Each form presents special difficulties with
the indirect discourse form being the most difficult. Some indirect discourse forms are among the most difficult syntactic forms
and are among the last learned by normal children (C. Chomsky,
1969).

DIRECT DISCOURSE

Virtually all reading materials used for reading instruction in
the primary grades use conversation as a general language format.
The direct discourse form is used to represent conversation in
these materials. It is used to such an extent that it is the single
most frequently used syntactic form in many of these materials
(Hargis, 1974).

Direct discourse forms are sentences which have transitive
verbs of a particular type which indicate that something is being
expressed. The complex objects of these transitive verbs are
duplicates of what was said. In print, this direct quote is contained within quotation marks and separated from the rest of
the sentence by a comma:

1. Mary said, "I want a puppy."
2. Jill said, "See the spotted puppy. I like it."

3. "I like the brown puppy," said Mary.
4. "How much are the puppies?" Jill asked.
5. "Three dollars," said Mr. Simms. "But for you, only one dollar."

More variation in word order is possible with the direct discourse form than in any other syntactic structure. In examples 1 and 2 the subject-verb-object word order is maintained. In example 3 we have an object-verb-subject order. In example 4 the order is object-subject-verb. Example 5 has a divided direct quote object with the order object-verb-subject-object.

Example 2 illustrates two sentences used as the direct quote object. Multiple sentences are often used in this manner in primary grade level reading materials.

The word order variation, the splitting of direct quote objects, and the use of multiple sentence objects constitute a considerable problem in dealing with the direct discourse form. In a study with hearing-impaired children, Hargis, Evans and Masters (1973) found that passages composed largely of direct discourse forms were significantly more difficult to comprehend than passages from the same book that were narrated without direct discourse use.

The transitive verb like *say* was the only verb used in four of the five examples. It is used with the greatest frequency in direct discourse. However, the transitive verb class which is used in direct discourse includes verbs such as *shout, whisper, cry, moaned, sobbed, exclaimed, admitted,* etc. These verbs carry additional meaning concerning the manner in which their direct quote objects are expressed.

Direct discourse forms in print do not mirror the conversation form which children are used to hearing. Also, the many variations of word order which are seen in print are not used frequently in speech. Probably the best way to introduce children to the printed representation of conversation is through the cartoon balloon format. Here the balloon leading to the lips of the actual speaker concretely bypasses the subject and *say* verb of the direct discourse form. The child sees who is talking. The artist's representation of the speaker can indicate concretely the manner in which the discourse is expressed. From this readiness base the child can be taken to the appropriate direct discourse forms which may be used to represent through print alone the context and conversation. The subject-verb-direct quote-object word order should be presented initially. Then altered word forms should be introduced carefully after these foundation concepts are mastered.

INDIRECT DISCOURSE

Indirect discourse has two primary syntactic forms. The conversational expression to be represented can take the infinitive form of a transitive verb complement or it can have a noun clause form. These two structures suggest the necessary readiness basis for indirect discourse. Children must understand both the infinitive form of transitive verb complements and noun clauses used as objects in simpler usages. Also, the direct discourse form provides an unaltered version of the discourse to be presented and it should precede the teaching of comparative indirect discourse structures. The following sentences illustrate the various forms of indirect discourse:

1. The boy said that he likes dogs.
2. Fred told Joe that he was in the fifth grade.
3. Pete told Fred who his teacher was.
4. Mary told Jill to get the book.
5. Mary asked Jill to get the hook.
6. Pete asked Fred who his teacher was.
7. Fred asked Joe if he liked school.
8. Fred asked Joe whether he liked school or not.
9. Pete told Fred what to take.
10. Pete asked Fred what to take.

There is a basic division among the transitive verb forms used in indirect discourse. The verb *tell* is used to relate declarative statements and commands while the verb *ask* is used to relate questions and requests. Verbs in the *say* class are used to relate declarative statements only. Example 1 illustrates the simplest noun clause form. Only declarative sentences may be embedded in the noun clause position following *say*. Examples 2 and 3 show noun clause objects of *tell*. Notice that the listeners in these indirect discourse examples appear as indirect objects. Only *say,* as in example 1, does not take this type indirect object.

Notice that the personal pronouns which appear in the subjects of the noun clauses (examples 1, 2, 3, 6, 7, 8) are changed from the first person forms of direct discourse. This change in form is a source of considerable difficulty both in comprehension and production for many children. Another problem which was noted by Carol Chomsky (1969) has to do with the proximity of the indirect object to these pronouns. She found a tendency for children to inappropriately interpret the referent of the pronoun in the noun clause as being the indirect object because of the close proximity.

Example 4 illustrates the indirect discourse form used to relate command or imperative sentences. Only the verb *tell* is used in this function. The command sentence is embedded as the transitive verb complement. The following examples illustrate the direct discourse (example 11) form and then the indirect discourse form (example 12).

11. The teacher said to Fred, "Sit down."
12. The teacher told Fred to sit down.

Example 5 illustrated the indirect discourse form used to relate requests. Only the verb *ask* can be used for this. The request sentence is embedded as a transitive verb complement in this form also. The request sentence can have the form of a yes/no question or an imperative sentence with the word *please* attached. The following examples show the two possible request sentences in direct discourse forms and then the single indirect discourse form.

13. Fred said, "Joe, will you help me."
14. Fred said, "Joe, help me, please."
15. Fred asked Joe to help him.

All questions either *wh* or yes/no appear as noun clauses following the verb *ask* in direct discourse. Carol Chomsky (1969) found that normal children tend to interpret *ask* as *tell* until quite late in the acquisition of these structures. This means that children often tend to mistakenly interpret as declarative sentences the questions embedded after *ask*. The following examples show the direct discourse and then the indirect discourse form for two different *wh* questions.

16. Joe said to Fred, "Where do you live?"
17. Joe asked Fred where he lived.
18. Mary said to Jill, "Who is your teacher?"
19. Mary asked Jill who her teacher was.

Yes/no questions embedded in indirect discourse forms are changed quite considerably from their actual conversational form. All yes/no questions will be introduced by *if* unless they contain the conjunction *or*. If *or* is used in the yes/no question, then it will be introduced by *whether*. These changes in structural appearance make these forms quite difficult to interpret. The following examples are direct and indirect forms of yes/no questions:

20. Joe said to Pete, "Do you like school?"
21. Joe asked Pete if he liked school.
22. Joe said to Pete, "Will you watch the football game or the baseball game?"
23. Joe asked Pete whether he would watch the football game or the baseball game.

In examples 9 and 10 the discourse is quite reduced. Both forms are question word noun clauses which have been further changed by the for/to transformation. Notice that even though the discourse in both sentences has been reduced to the identical phrase *what to take,* the phrase represents a command in sentence 9 and a *wh* question in sentence 10. Comprehension of such structures requires mastery of the distinction between *ask* and *tell* as well as the ability to recover the information which has been deleted from the discourse sentences.

SUMMARY

Direct and indirect discourse forms comprise a very difficult set of structures. Teaching direct discourse forms in print can be related meaningfully to the cartoon balloon format for representing conversation. Teaching indirect discourse forms can be concretely tied to the simpler direct discourse forms. The ask/tell distinction can be developed by using *ask* with such question types in direct discourse, then illustrating the structural changes made in the transfer to indirect discourse.

EXERCISES

Change the following direct discourse sentences to indirect discourse:

1. The lady said, "My dog is sick."

   The lady said that her dog is sick.

2. Mother asked, "Did the boy leave?"

   Mother asked if the boy left.

3. The doctor asked the nurse, "Are you going to the hospital or home?"

   The doctor asked the nurse whether she was going to the hospital or home.

4. The lady asked, "Where is the library?"

   The lady asked where the library is.

5. "Go home," Joe said to Fred.

   Joe told Fred to go home.

CHAPTER 32

WORD ORDER TRANSFORMATIONS

CHANGES IN NORMAL word order pose significant comprehension difficulties to children who are in the developmental process of language acquisition. There are a number of word order transformations that do not change the essential meaning of sentences but which have considerable affect on the structural appearance of them. The purpose of this chapter is to identify the most common forms of word order changes in sentences which have not been covered in prior chapters.

VERB PHRASE MOVEMENT

This transformation occurs in conjoined sentences. The verb phrase of the second sentence is moved to the front of that sentence. In the following examples the first sentence shows the structure before the word order transformation.

1. Joe plans to go, and he will go.
   Joe plans to go, and go he will.

Not all conjoined sentences will transform in this manner. In order to be transformed in this fashion the first conjoined sentence should express intent and the second should show affirmation.

NEGATIVE MOVEMENT

This transformation occurs with sentences containing negative words such as never, seldom or rarely.

1. She had never seen such a large house.
   Never had she seen such a large house.
2. The children seldom have much fun at school.
   Seldom do the children have much fun at school.

In these structures negative words move to the front of the sentence and the sentence takes on the structural form of a yes/no question.

ADVERB OF PLACE MOVEMENT

In this transformation the adverb of place may be moved to the beginning of the sentence. In some sentences one additional movement may occur and this is the shift of the subject to the position following the verb.

1. The puppy ran up the stairs.
   Up the stairs the puppy ran.
   Up the stairs ran the puppy.

2. A picture of Santa hangs on my wall.
   On my wall a picture of Santa hangs.
   On my wall hangs a picture of Santa.

MOVEMENT AROUND BE

When the auxiliary of a sentence contains *be+ing*, the verb phrase may be moved to the front of the sentence and the subject to the end.

1. Joe was leaning on a tree.
   Leaning on a tree was Joe.

2. The children were walking to school.
   Walking to school were the children.

DIRECT QUOTE MOVEMENT

Some of the movement possible in direct discourse sentence forms was discussed in the last chapter. They are quite probably subject to more word order change than any other sentence type. Notice that the subject, verb and direct quote object of the following sentence may be placed in any position.

1. Joe said, "I like candy."
   "I like candy," said Joe.
   "I like candy," Joe said.
   Said Joe, "I like candy."

OBJECT MOVEMENT

The object noun phrases of transitive verb sentences are occasionally moved to the beginning of those sentences. This is apparently done to focus more attention on the object.

1. You should see that movie.
   That movie you should see.

2. He fixed the motor quickly.
   The motor he fixed quickly.

Noun clauses used as objects may move in this same fashion.
3. I think it is a dog.
   It is a dog, I think.

CONCLUSION

The altered word order which was described in this chapter may change the difficulty of sentences to a great extent without changing meaning significantly. The purpose of most of these transformations seems to be to add emphasis or focus more attention on certain sentence parts. Word order changes like these have a high rate of occurrence in beginning reading material and children's literature. For this reason these structural changes may pose a considerable problem for many children.

An extensive treatment on word order transformations is provided by Hooper and Thompson (1973).

ASSESSMENT PROCEDURES

A NECESSARY BASIS for assessing any child's level of language functioning are test items and procedures which represent the scope of language structures. The previous chapters have outlined what the author believes to be the most essential elements of English syntactic structures. In this chapter the purpose is to describe methods of assessing a child's comprehension of syntactic structures.

Adequate assessment identifies what the child knows of the scope of syntactic structures, but further, this assessment relates this knowledge to the point or points in a developmental sequence. Identification of position in this sequence indicates what the child should be introduced to next and what constitutes the child's readiness base from which the clinician may work. The developmental sequence was discussed to some extent in each chapter. However, in reality, language is not acquired segmentally by such categories, but it is more likely that acquisition is progressing to some extent cross-categorically and simultaneously.

COMPREHENSION

The emphasis throughout the book has been more on comprehension of syntactic structures than on their production. The assessment techniques which will be discussed will also focus on comprehension. One of the main problems in assessing the comprehension of various syntactic structures is to do so without having the child use production skills.

Growth in comprehension ability exceeds production ability. It is, therefore, of quite limited value to use assessment techniques which rely only on language production data for insight concerning the specific structures children may comprehend. This is especially true for younger children. This is not to say that production and its assessment are not important. The assessment of the production of syntax has a separate focus and poses a distinct set of problems.

PROCEDURES

Object manipulation in response to text items is an effective way of assessing comprehension without requiring a verbal response.

Amy Sheldon (1972) studied the comprehension of relative clauses in children three to five years of age. She chose to test comprehension by means of a toy-moving task. The children used toy animals to act out action sequences described in sentences containing various types of relative clauses. For example, the child would be given a sentence like "The cow that the bird stands on bumps into the dog." The child would move the toy cow, bird and dog according to his or her comprehension of the sentence. The examiner would note each moving response that the child made, either correct or incorrect. She points out a number of advantages for toy-moving tasks. These tasks provided a record of mistakes as well as correct responses. There is a much lower probability of doing them correctly by chance than for tasks such as multiple choice picture identification. It is often possible to identify the correct picture without having understood all or even part of the tested sentence. Also, a considerable advantage of using toys is that children enjoy making them do things and toys will hold their attention. Sheldon found that four trial examples were sufficient to teach normal children in this age group the format for this type test.

Other object manipulation tasks may require little teaching time. In the author's experiments in assessing certain determiner structures, blocks and small shoe boxes were used. The items here were "put a block in each of the boxes," "Put a block in every box." With a combination of blocks and balls the directions were "Put all of the blocks in the box," "Put some of the balls in the box." The focus of attention in each test sentence was the determiner structures *a, each of, every, all of* and *some of*. In tasks such as these the particular structures under consideration are embedded in imperative sentences. The child must understand these *vehicle* sentences already or they must be learned before this kind of test can be validly conducted. Whenever a syntactic structure to be assessed is embedded in another sentence or structure, it is essential that this vehicle sentence or structure be familiar. Imperative sentences and question forms are frequently used as such vehicles. Care must be taken to find whether or not they are familiar before they should be considered for use in assessment.

Another major consideration for constructing test items to assess syntax is that the vocabulary used in them must be familiar. Otherwise the child may miss an item because of an unknown noun, verb or adjective rather than the lack of comprehension of the syntactic forms which contain them. It is necessary to assess knowledge of the vocabulary used in the test in isolation or in quite simple sentence frames as a pretest condition. This is probably best accomplished by multiple choice picture selection tests over the specific vocabulary in question.

Some syntactic forms lend themselves to multiple choice picture selection. If it is a choice of only two pictures, then several items should be included to reduce the likelihood of chance in the selection of the correct picture. With younger children it is probably better to use only two pictures for the multiple choice response. Figures 1, 2 and 3 show some possible formats.

Pictures or objects may be used to assess certain syntactic forms embedded in yes/no questions. Though a verbal response is necessary, a minimum of production skill is required to make a yes or no response. Again, since only two responses are possible, several items of this type should be used to confirm the reliability of responses. Also, the child must understand the appropriate yes/no questions before they may be used in assessment. Figures 4, 5 and 6 show test items of this type.

All syntactic forms do not lend themselves to assessment through any single format. Therefore it is necessary to mix the format to get the best one for each structure.

Carol Chomsky (1969) used an interview technique in assessing acquisition of syntax in children from five to ten. This approach requires the most extensive use of a child's language production ability. This technique is appropriate for children who have functional language comparable to that of a normal child of four or five. At this level most children will be amenable to answering questions, cooperating in carrying out tasks, and playing games. Only the more complex syntactic structures would be assessed, but it would still be necessary to control the directions and questions conveying the test items to within the basal comprehension level of each child. In assessing a child's comprehension of *ask* and *tell* constructions, C. Chomsky used requests and imperative statements such as "Will you ask X what time it is?" "Tell X how many toys there are here." "Ask X what to put in the box." "Tell X to come back." "Ask X to go back to class." It is obvious that the comprehension check for these items is the production of sentences. However, at this level of assessment this approach seems quite appropriate.

Severely hearing-impaired children may require several adjustments in the mode of communicating the test items. The items should be repeated as often as need be to make sure the child is not making an incorrect response because of not perceiving all elements in the items. For older children the simplest adjustment is to give the test items through print, or through print and other communication modes. If speech is used, then appropriate attention to amplification may be important. If the child has manual communication skill, then the test may be administered through signs and finger spelling. Here again the sign vocabulary should be familiar to the child. The syntactic components should be finger spelled to insure correspondence to English.

CONCLUSION

In assessing comprehension of syntactic structures, several conditions were emphasized. One was the careful control of the use of vocabulary. It is necessary to use already known vocabulary in the structures being assessed. Also, if the structures are embedded in other sentences or structures, they must be familiar to the child. Additionally, it is important to make sure that the test directions are mastered and that they are not changed indiscriminately or abruptly during the test.

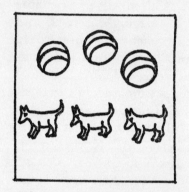 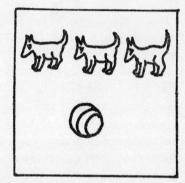

Figure 1. The structure being assessed here is the comparative form *as many . . . as*. The examiner says, "Point to the picture that has as many balls as dogs." In this item the comparative is embedded in both a relative clause and in an imperative sentence.

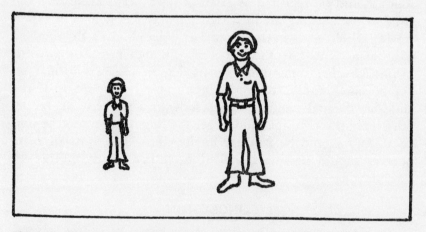

Figure 2. The structure being assessed here is the comparative prearticle *the taller of*. The examiner says, "Point to the taller of the two boys." In this item an imperative sentence is used.

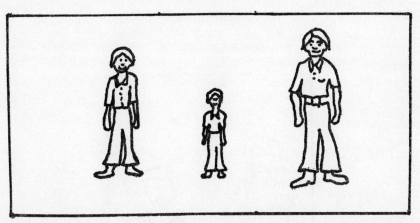

Figure 3. The structure under consideration in this item is the superlative prearticle *shortest of*. The examiner says, "Point to the shortest of the boys." The superlative is in an imperative sentence.

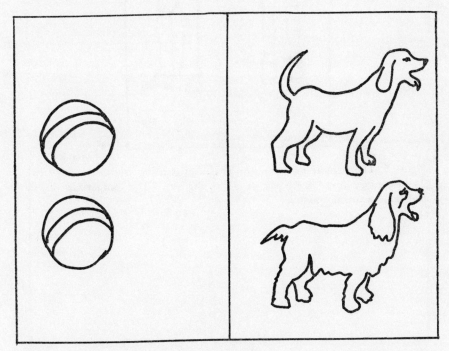

Figure 4. The comparative structure *as many . . . as* is being assessed in this item. The examiner says, "Are there as many balls as there are dogs?" The comparative form is embedded in a yes/no question.

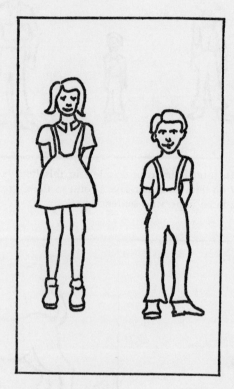

Figure 5. The comparative structure *as* . . . *as* is being assessed in this item. The examiner says, "Is the boy as tall as the girl?" The comparative is embedded in a yes/no question.

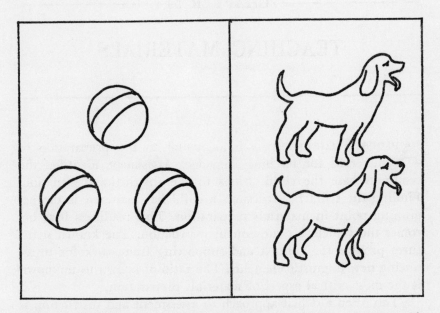

Figure 6. The comparative structure *more . . . than* is being assessed in this item. The examiner says, "Are there more balls than there are dogs?" The comparative is embedded in a yes/no question.

TEACHING MATERIALS

A DEQUATE ASSESSMENT is fundamental to the preparation of materials for teaching language. Assessment identifies the readiness base the child brings to the instructional situation. Finding the syntactic structures a child has mastered is the beginning point in materials preparation. This readiness base becomes the vehicle for subsequent instruction. The known structures provide the context and supporting framework for introducing new linguistic elements. The ratio of known to unknown is the most critical aspect of materials preparation.

Too often a deficit approach to assessment and instruction is used. Here, the focus of instruction is on what a child does not know. The child's deficits and weaknesses may have been precisely identified, but little attention is given to identifying what he knows so that a comfortable basis for instruction can be prepared. Children are often inundated with instruction on unfamiliar or strange items. This approach can be highly frustrating and is often failure inducing.

INSTRUCTIONAL RATIOS

Of fundamental importance to language instruction is the ratio of known to unknown elements. Materials that are appropriately prepared with sufficient familiar content are attention maintaining. Children will have sufficient familiar context to assist them in coping with the newly introduced unfamiliar components. The children can maintain attention because the material provides enough context so that they can stay on task. Appropriately prepared materials are also reinforcing because children find that they can comprehend them and they are able to stay on task. Emmett Betts (1946) formalized some ratios for the purpose of identifying reading materials which were suitable for reading instruction for individual children. In general, he stated that in reading material fewer than 5 percent of the total running words could be unfamiliar. If the percentage of unfamiliar words was in the range of 2 to 5 percent, then the child could maintain a comprehension level of 75 percent. Comprehension falls off rapidly when this percentage is exceeded.

This ratio of knowns to unknowns has proven to be effective in preparing connected language activities and materials for handicapped children also. However, more than just unfamiliar printed words must be considered. Syntactic structures, vocabulary and figurative forms all may require attention. For drill and seatwork activities this ratio may be adjusted somewhat, but the 75 percent comprehension level must be maintained. Usually this is accomplished by making sure that at least 75 percent of the individual drill items are familiar. If this general guideline is followed, drill work can be attention maintaining and reinforcing.

At beginning levels of language instruction, the child may have a quite limited range of familiar language structures. At this level the appropriate ratios may be maintained by heavy repetition of the known elements. Otherwise the familiar component should be supplied by nonlinguistic contextual support such as pictures.

The following selections illustrate the controlled use of context, both linguistic and pictorial. The unfamiliar structure being introduced in the first story is *too—for—too*. The second story introduces *so—that*. These structures were discussed in the chapter on cause and effect. The familiar linguistic context is limited primarily to simple sentences plus possessives, indirect objects, the negative transformation and intensifiers.

Most commercially prepared basal reading material should not be used with language handicapped children. Even though the basal readers do control the introduction rate for unfamiliar printed words, they do not control the introduction of syntactic or figurative structures. In a recent study of the primers and first

TOO BIG FOR BOB

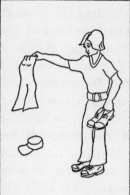

Bob has a brother. Bob's brother is big. His name is Joe. Joe gave Bob some clothes

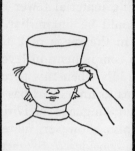

Joe gave Bob a hat. The hat covers Bob's eyes. The hat is very big. The hat is too big for Bob to wear.

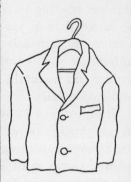

Joe gave Bob a coat. The coat covers Bob's hands. The coat is very big. The coat is too big for Bob to wear.

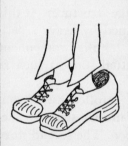

Joe gave Bob shoes. The shoes are very big. The shoes are too big for Bob to wear.

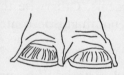

Joe gave Bob pants. The pants cover Bob's feet. The pants are very big. The pants are too big for Bob to wear.

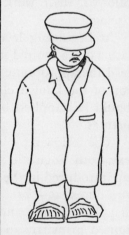

Bob looked funny. Joe laughed.

BEEZER AT THE BEACH

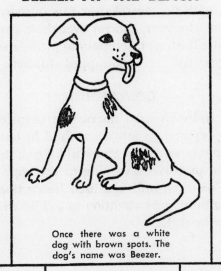

Once there was a white dog with brown spots. The dog's name was Beezer.

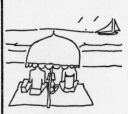

One day the family took Beezer to the beach. The sun was very hot. The sun was so hot that the family sat under the beach umbrella.

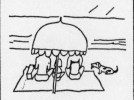

Beezer wanted to sit under the umbrella. It was very crowded. It was so crowded that Beezer could not sit under the umbrella.

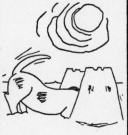

Beezer crawled into a sand castle. The castle was very small. The castle was so small that it fell.

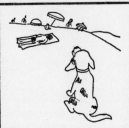

The beach was very crowded. It was so crowded that Beezer got lost. It was so crowded that Beezer could not find the family.

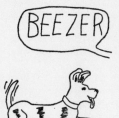

Soon Beezer heard the family call him. The family found Beezer.

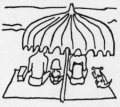

The next day the family bought a new beach umbrella. It was very big. The umbrella was so big that Beezer could sit under it. The whole family sat under the umbrella.

readers (Hargis, 1974) virtually all syntactic structures were found in them with no control over this introduction or subsequent repetition. However, control over these structures is often the most critical adjustment necessary to provide suitable reading and language material for handicapped children.

CONCLUSION

Adequately individualized instruction requires that the material which is prepared for any given child be based on information gained from assessment of that child. From this information, material may be prepared according to the appropriate instructional ratios. Too often individualized instruction is thought of as simply giving individual attention to a child without regard to the material for the child.

BIBLIOGRAPHY

Akmajian, Adrian: On deriving cleft sentences from pseudocleft sentences. *Linguistic Inquiry, 1*:149, 1970.

Betts, Emmett Albert: *Foundation of Reading Instruction.* New York, Am. Bk, 1946.

Bolinger, Dwight: *The Phrasal Verb in English.* Cambridge, Harvard U Pr, 1971.

Bresnan, Joan W.: Syntax of the comparative clause construction in English. *Linguistic Inquiry, 4*:275, 1973.

Bresnan, Joan W.: Comparative deletion and constraints on transformations. *Linguistic Analysis, 1*:25, 1975.

Brown, R., and Bellugi, U.: Three processes in child's acquisition of syntax. In Lenneberg, Eric (Ed.): *New Directions in the Studies of Language.* Cambridge, MIT Press, 1964.

Brown, Roger: *Social Psychology.* New York, Free Pr, 1965.

Brown, R., and Hanlon, C.: Derivational complexities and the order of acquisition in child speech. In Hayes, J. R. (Ed.): *Cognition and the Development of Language.* New York, Wiley, 1970.

Chomsky, Carol: *The Acquisition of Syntax of Children from 5 to 10.* Cambridge, MIT Press, 1969.

Chomsky, Noam: *Syntactic Structures.* The Hague, Mouton, 1957.

Chomsky, Noam: *Aspects of the Theory of Syntax.* Cambridge, MIT Press, 1965.

Curtiss, Susan, Fromkin, V., Krashen, S., Rigler, D., and Rigler, M.: The linguistic development of Genie. *Language, 50*:528, 1974.

Fries, Charles C.: *American English Grammar.* New York, Appleton, 1940.

Furth, Hans G.: *Thinking Without Language.* New York, Free Pr, 1966.

Hakutani, Yoshinobu, and Hargis, Charles H.: The syntax of modal constructions in English. *Lingua, 30*:301, 1972.

Hargis, Charles H.: The relationship of available instructional reading materials to deficiency in reading achievement. *Am Ann Deaf, 115*:27, 1970.

Hargis, Charles H., and Ahlersmeyer, D.: The significance of grammar in teaching arithmetic to educable retarded children. *Education and Training of the Mentally Retarded, 5*:104, 1970.

Hargis, Charles H.: The significance of the grammar of one-to-one correspondence in teaching counting to the retarded. *Education and Training of the Mentally Retarded, 6*:170, 1971.

215

Hargis, Charles H.: Cause and Effect. Paper presented at the summer meeting of the Linguistic Society of America, July 29, 1972.

Hargis, Charles H., Evans, Carole C., and Masters, Carolyn: A criticism of the direct discourse form in primary level basal readers. *The Volta Review, 75:*557, 1973.

Hargis, Charles H.: An analysis of the syntactic and figurative structure of popular first grade level basal readers. Paper presented at the 12th Southeastern Conference on Linguistics, November 1, 1974.

Hargis, Charles H., and Lamm, Carolyn O.: Have and be: A lexicon of verb forms. *The Volta Review, 76:*420, 1974.

Hargis, Charles H.: Just, even, and only: a lexicon of modifiers. *The Volta Review, 77:*368, 1975a.

Hargis, Charles H.: The syntax of comparative constructions and mathematical reasoning. *Teaching English to the Deaf, 2:*17, 1975b.

Hargis, Charles H.: A linguistic outline of cause and effect. *Teaching English to the Deaf, 2:*16, 1975c.

Hargis, Charles H., Mercaldo, David J., and Johnson, H. Wayne: A linguistic and cognitive perspective on retardation. *J Genet Psychol, 126:*145, 1975d.

Hooper, Joan B., and Thompson, Sandra A.: On the applicability of root transformations. *Linguistic Inquiry, 4:*465, 1973.

Jespersen, Otto: *Essentials of English Grammar*. London, George Allen and Unwin, 1933.

Klima, Edward S.: Negation in English. In Fodor, Jerry A., and Katz, Jerrold J. (Eds.): *The Structure of Language,* Englewood Cliffs, P-H, 1964.

Lees, Robert B.: *The Grammar of English Nominalizations*. The Hague, Mouton, 1963.

Lenneberg, Eric H.: *Biological Foundations of Language*. New York, Wiley, 1967.

Lester, Mark: *Introductory Transformational Grammar of English*. New York, HR & W, 1971.

Makkai, Adam: *Idiom Structure in English*. The Hague, Mouton, 1972.

McNeill, David: Developmental Psycholinguistics. In Smith, Frank, and Miller, George A. (Eds.): *The Genesis of Language*. Cambridge, MIT Press, 1966.

McNeill, David: *The Acquisition of Language*. New York, Har Row, 1970.

Menyuk, Paula: Syntactic rules used by children from preschool through first grade. *Child Devel, 35:*533, 1964.

Menyuk, Paula: *Sentences Children Use*. Cambridge, MIT Press, 1969.

Nilsen, Don Lee Fred: *English Abverbials*. The Hargue, Mouton, 1972.

Palermo, David S., and Molfese, Dennis L.: Language acquisition from age five onward. *Psychol Bull, 78:*409, 1972.

Piaget, Jean: Language and intellectual operations. In Furth, Hans G.: *Piaget and Knowledge*. Englewood Cliffs, P-H, 1969, pp. 121-130.

Power, D. J., and Quigley, S. P.: Deaf children's acquisition of the passive voice, *J Speech Hear Res, 16:*5, 1973.

Quigley, S. P., Smith, N. L., and Wilbur, R. B.: Comprehension of relativized sentences by deaf students. *J Speech Hear Res, 17:*325, 1974.

Quigley, S. P., Wilbur, R. B., and Montanelli, D. S.: Question formation in the langauge of deaf students. *J Speech Hear Res, 17:*699, 1974.

Schreiber, Peter A.: Some constraints on the formation of English sentence adverbs. *Linguistic Inquiry, 2:*83, 1971.

Sheldon, Amy: The Role of Parallel Function in the Acquisition of Relative Clauses. Paper presented at the Forty-Seventh Annual Meeting of the Linguistic Society of America, December 27, 1972.

Streng, Alice: *Syntax Speech and Hearing.* New York, Grune, 1972.

Wilbur, R. B., Quigley, S. P., and Montanelli, D. S.: Conjoined structures in the language of deaf students. *J Speech Hear Res, 18:*319, 1975.

Zwickey, Arnold M., and Zwickey, Ann: How come and what for. *Ohio State University Working Papers in Linguistics,* No. 8, 1971, pp. 174-185.

INDEX